TAKING CHARGE

of Arthritis

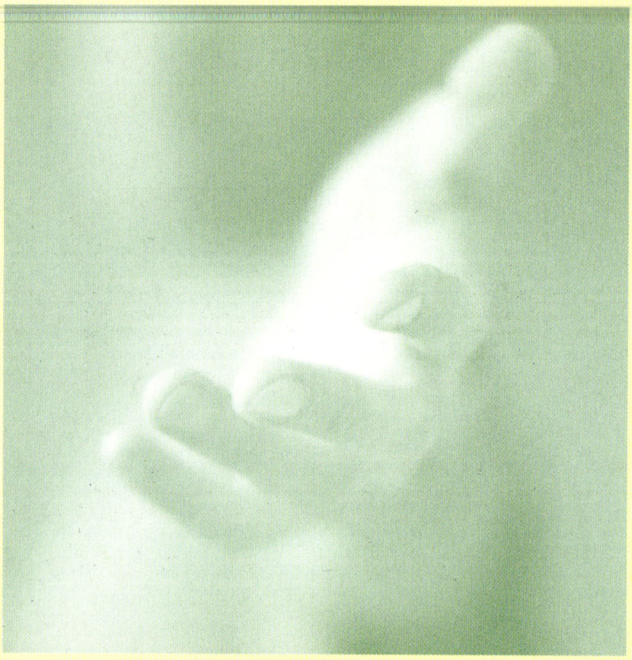

TAKING CHARGE of Arthritis

Larry Katzenstein

The Reader's Digest Association, Inc.
Pleasantville, New York/Montreal

Contents

CHAPTER 5

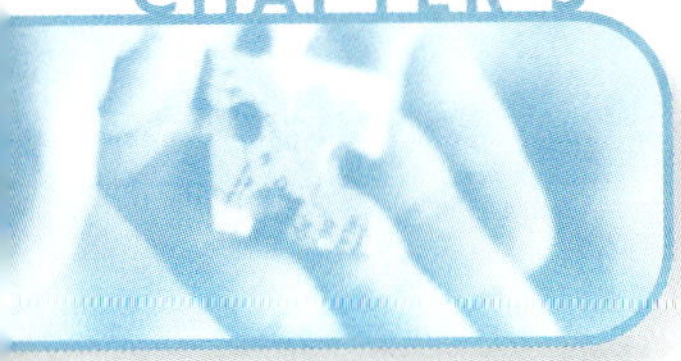

CHAPTER 6

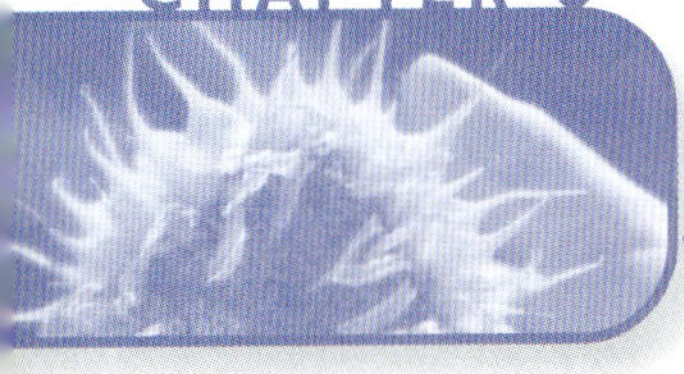

CHAPTER 7

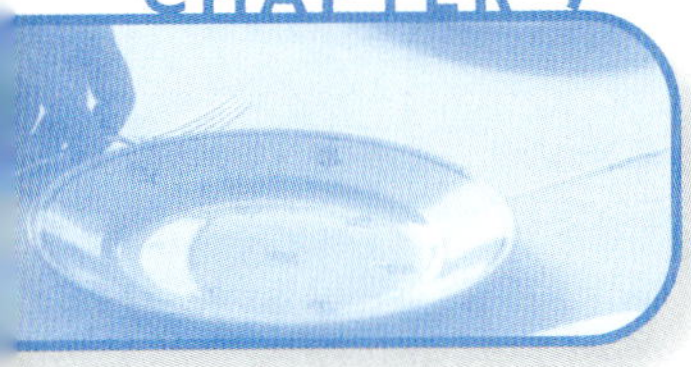

CHAPTER 8

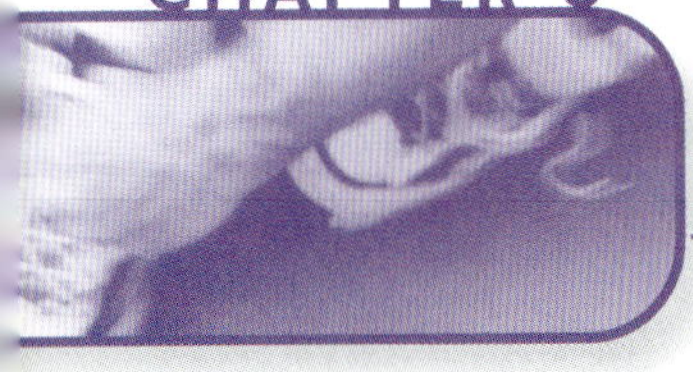

Reader's Digest Project Staff

Editorial Director
Wayne Kalyn

Production Technology Manager
Douglas A. Croll

Editorial Manager
Christine R. Guido

Contributors

Writer
Larry Katzenstein

Design
Spinning Egg Design Group

Senior Designer
Martha Grossman

Illustrators
Articulate Graphics, Hugo Cruz, Linda Frichtell

Indexer
Robert Elwood

Medical Consultants

Eddys Disla, MD
Associate chief of rheumatology, Cabrini Medical Center, New York, and a fellow of the American College of Rheumatology

Dr. John Hassall, F.R.A.C.P., emeritus consultant in rheumatology at the Royal Prince Alfred Hospital, Sydney, Australia

Reader's Digest Health Publishing

Senior Vice President
Thomas Gardner

Vice President/Publisher
Shirrel Rhoades

Marketing
Edith Berelson

US 4011/H-US

Reader's Digest Illustrated Reference Books

Editor-in-Chief
Christopher Cavanaugh

Art Director
Joan Mazzeo

Operations Manager
William J. Cassidy

Library of Congress Cataloging in Publication Data

Taking charge of arthritis: an action guide to managing your health and well-being.
p. cm.
Includes index.
ISBN 0-7621-0322-1 (hardcover)
ISBN 0-7621-0344-2 (paperback)
1. Arthritis—Popular works. I. Reader's Digest Association.

RC933 .T27 2001
616.7122—dc21 00-068429

Address any comments about *Taking Charge of Arthritis* to:
Reader's Digest
Editor-in-Chief, Illustrated Reference Books
Reader's Digest Road
Pleasantville, NY 10570

To order additional copies of *Taking Charge of Arthritis*, call 1-800-846-2100

Visit our website at www.readersdigest.com

Printed in the United States of America

1 3 5 7 9 10 8 6 4 2

Note to Readers

The information in this book should not be substituted for, or used to alter, medical therapy without your doctor's advice. For a specific health problem, consult your physician for guidance.

About This Book

If you gathered the horde of arthritis books that have been published and stacked them up in your living room, you would be justified in asking why READER'S DIGEST is bothering to publish one more on a topic that has been written about ad infinitum. Clearly, a reader can get a king's ransom of information from the vast library already devoted to the condition.

Well, maybe not. *Taking Charge of Arthritis* contains the latest, most relevant information about managing and preventing arthritis and—here is the real kicker—supplies you with practical advice and strategies to use that information to your benefit. In a nutshell, it is news you can use. If your goal is to treat, prevent, or overcome the chronic pain of osteoarthritis or its fiery cousin, rheumatoid arthritis, this volume will give you the facts, the plan, and the inspiration to accomplish it.

The book is, to steal a line from those old breath-mint commercials, two books in one. If you are the type of person who likes to follow a program, *Taking Charge of Arthritis* has come up with a very successful one for you. Based on the Arthritis Self-Help Course pioneered by Stanford University and taught across the country by the Arthritis Foundation, our program will supply you with the steps and motivation to overcome your pain and disability and to lead a richer, fuller life.

On the other hand, if you are the type of person who is allergic to programs and who prefers to pick and choose what's right for you, this book will work like a charm. You will find information on virtually every facet of arthritis that you can use today, helping you achieve a measure of freedom from your condition tomorrow and into the future.

Whether it be that new arthritis drug, the new alternative therapy that the newspapers and TV news shows are all talking about, or the highly effective time-proven benefits of losing weight and getting exercise, *Taking Charge of Arthritis* has you covered.

If you have arthritis and have been focusing on coping with your condition, it is time to raise your sights. You can control your arthritis—to a greater degree than you imagined.

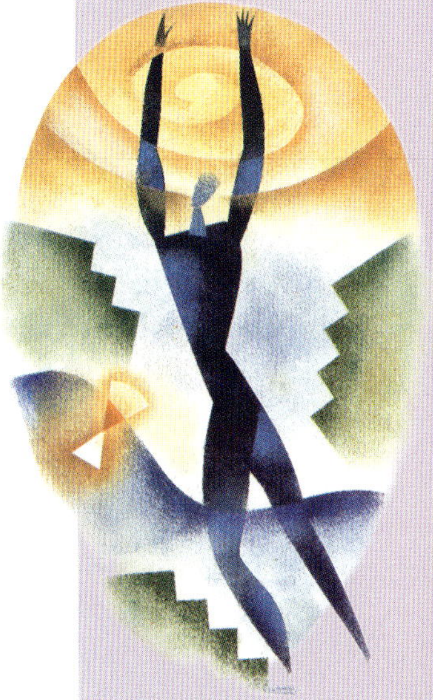

Foreword

These are exciting times in the treatment of arthritis. Never before have so many treatment options been available to the patient. We physicians often have many approaches to attack the arthritis process, but it is well-informed patients who are best able to take advantage of them: they ask the right questions in the doctor's office, they know when to call the doctor when a treatment isn't working out, and they are willing to learn more about their condition and the new treatments available.

I can tell during the first visit to my office which patients are more likely to do well: they are usually the ones motivated to learn about their illness. These patients often are suffering from severe arthritis, but they are not willing to give up. They assess the situation and look, along with their doctors, for the right treatment for them. There is overwhelming evidence that educated patients do better—not only with arthritis, but with most diseases.

I know that dealing with arthritis can be frustrating and challenging. It causes people to get angry, it causes people to isolate themselves, it causes people to become depressed. *Taking Charge of Arthritis* is a valuable help for all arthritis sufferers, empowering the unmotivated patient and further empowering the patient who is already on the self-care road. This easy-to-use but authoritative book provides you with the latest information, practical methods to channel it into your life, and the motivation to do so.

I firmly believe that education—getting all the facts—is the foundation of planned success in achieving just about anything: baseball players do it when they study "batting tapes" to help them get out of a slump, politicians do it when preparing for a debate to help them get an edge on their opponent. The patient who is trying to get her life back from arthritis should approach the disease in the exact same way. With *Taking Charge of Arthritis* in your hands, you have no excuse not to.

We are living in the Information Age. An explosion of information is available on the Internet, with its numerous health-oriented sites. Unfortunately, time, patience, and a healthy skepticism are required while sifting through the information on the 'net. Not with *Taking Charge of Arthritis*. The information is accurate, accessible, reliable.

There are few conditions that affect your life in such an intense way as arthritis. Things that you used to do without even thinking about them, such as brushing your teeth, getting dressed, or even feeding yourself, now become major challenges. After all, our joints work for us silently and effectively, enabling us not only to move around and use tools but also to express ourselves in every possible way: from painting and knitting to singing and talking (which depend on our jaw and larynx joints working together).

Conquering arthritis means staying active and participating in as many everyday activities as possible. This is best accomplished when we know what to expect from the disease and how to deal with it. One patient I feel very proud of has done just that. She is a 50-year-old woman with rheumatoid arthritis. She has been on prednisone, methotrexate, cyclosporin, hydroxychloroquine, etanercept. She also had her knee joints replaced, and has even suffered a pulmonary embolism.

And guess what? She remains active, holds down a full-time job, walks without a limp, and her hands are free of any noticeable deformity after more than 10 years of severe arthritis. She tries to give me credit for her happy outcome, but I know (and tell her all the time) that it takes two to tango: a caring doctor and an educated patient who has a grasp on every facet of arthritis. –Eddys Disla, MD

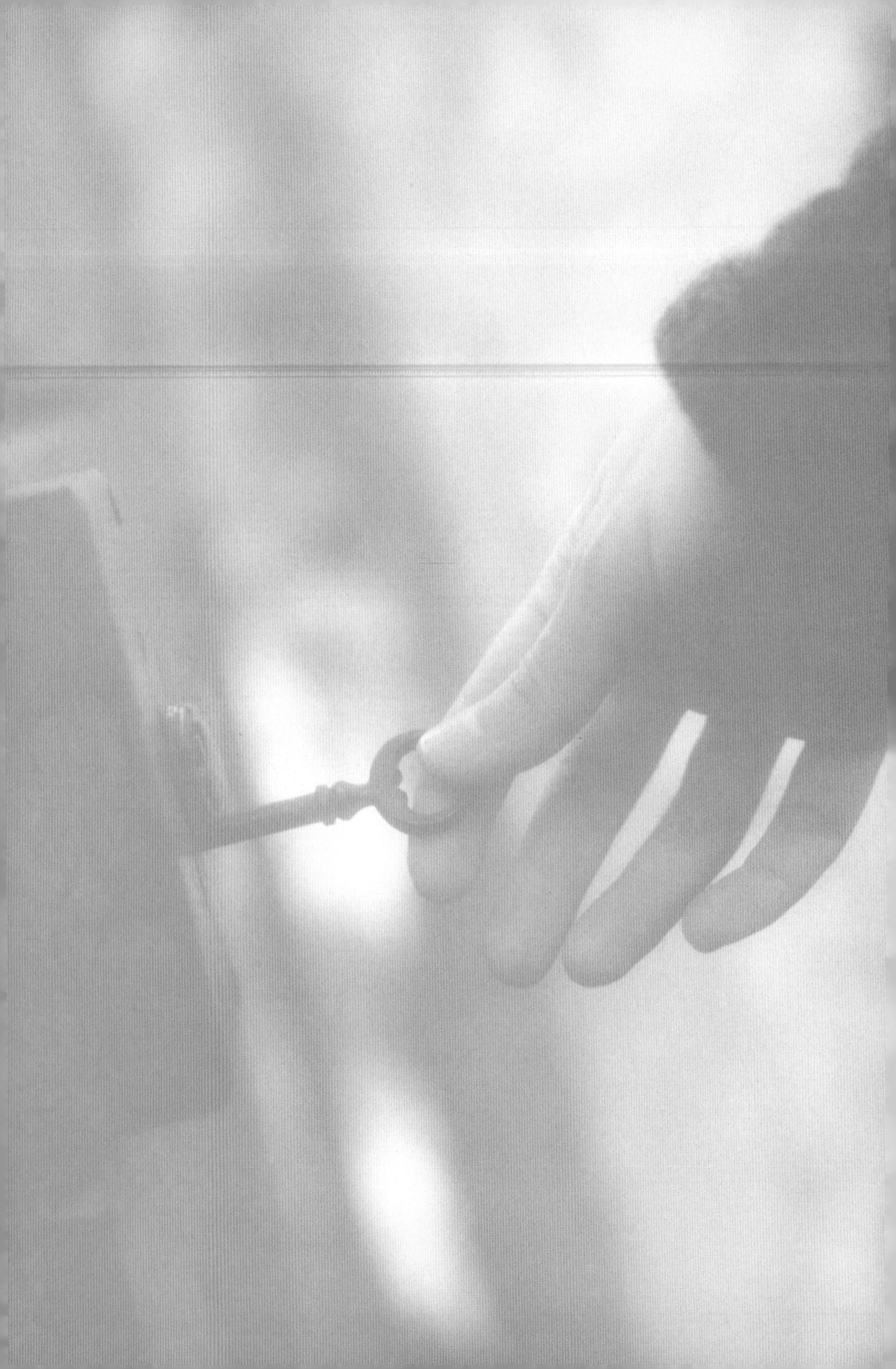

1 Confronting the Problem

If you have arthritis... and have been focusing mainly on coping with your condition... it's time to raise your sights, because you're capable of doing much better. You can control your arthritis—to a much greater degree than you've ever imagined.

KEY CONCEPT

Self-Empowerment: The belief in your ability to organize and devise a course of action that will result in mastering a situation. In short, controlling your own destiny.

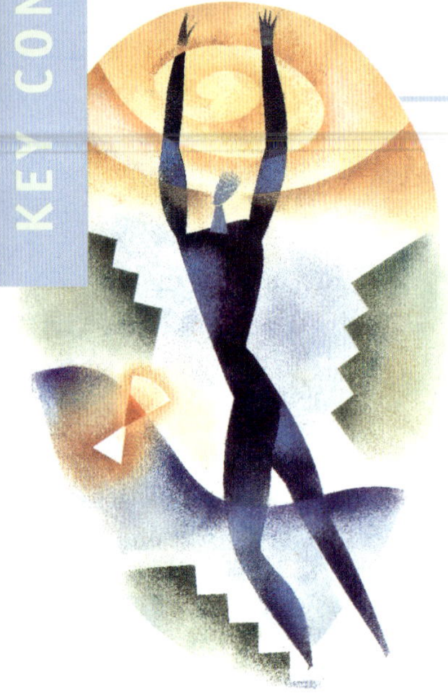

Attitude Is (Almost) Everything

Since arthritis is a chronic disease, many patients resign themselves to a "life sentence" of painful joints and the disability they can cause. Such a defeatist attitude practically guarantees that you won't get better and may get a lot worse—because when it comes to arthritis, mind really does matter.

The confidence to overcome. Thousands of people who suffer from arthritis have discovered a simple yet powerful truth that can provide hope and strength to just about anyone who develops the condition: The most successful patients, the ones who go on to live richer, fuller lives, are the ones who are most confident they can overcome the limitations of their disease. Researchers have studied many patients enrolled in arthritis self-help programs to find out what behavioral changes are most important. Much to their surprise, the researchers found that successfully overcoming symptoms hinged mainly on patients' confidence that they could.

What's more, a positive attitude was even more important to a patient's success than following her doctor's advice on treatment, nutrition, or exercise. This mindset—the conviction that you control your destiny—is called self-empowerment.

Defeating Arthritis = Knowledge + Action

In *Taking Charge of Arthritis*, you'll learn everything you need to know about your condition—from the newest information

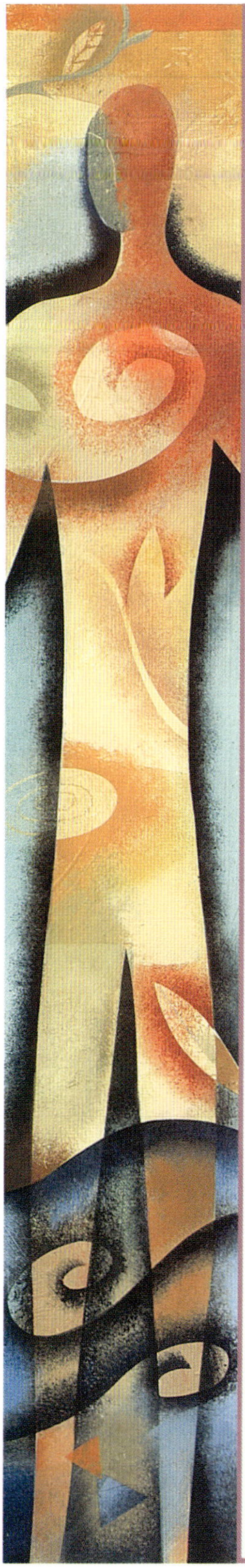

REAL-LIFE MEDICINE

Living with Osteoarthritis

Susan Louer, a retired New York City teacher, learned how to take charge of her arthritis by enrolling in the Arthritis Self-Help Course sponsored by the Arthritis Foundation. She found the course so helpful that she now teaches it to others. Here's what she says about her take-charge approach to her condition:

"I signed up for the course about five years after developing osteoarthritis of the knee. I wanted to know more about arthritis, and since I knew this was a chronic illness, I wanted to find the best ways of dealing with it.

> **"...It's up to you to make things better..."**

"Having arthritis is very hard, because you know it's forever—it's not going to go away. The course shows you that a positive, affirmative attitude about arthritis can really help you take charge of it. You realize that it's up to you to make things better for yourself and that there are some very effective things you can do to control your arthritis rather than let it control you.

"One of the most important things I learned was the value of setting short-term goals. Just pick one realistic goal for the week—walking for 10 minutes without stopping, for example. Then you decide when you're going to do it and how often.

"I've incorporated much of what I've learned in the course into my life. For example, I've gotten meditation into my mornings and find it's very helpful for relaxation. I also exercise regularly, every day if possible, doing stretching exercises as well as ones to strengthen my hamstring and quadriceps muscles.

"I've also learned to cope with the ups and downs that arthritis hands you. Sometimes you're going along just fine—you may not even be thinking about arthritis or even remember you have it—then all of a sudden you put your foot down on a step or get up from a chair, and you know things are going to be different for the next month.

"But when arthritis flares, you learn to adjust. You know it'll take you more time to get going in the morning so you wake up earlier, or you avoid the steps in the subway by taking the bus instead. You learn to plan, to take charge, and that way you can greatly improve the quality of your life."

about causes to the latest breakthroughs in conventional and alternative treatments. But even more important, you'll learn to become an effective practitioner of self-empowerment. You'll do that by formulating an effective arthritis action plan that incorporates the eight strategies for taking control of your condition.

BONING UP: Arthritis is often thought of as a problem of old age. But nearly three of every five patients are under age 65.

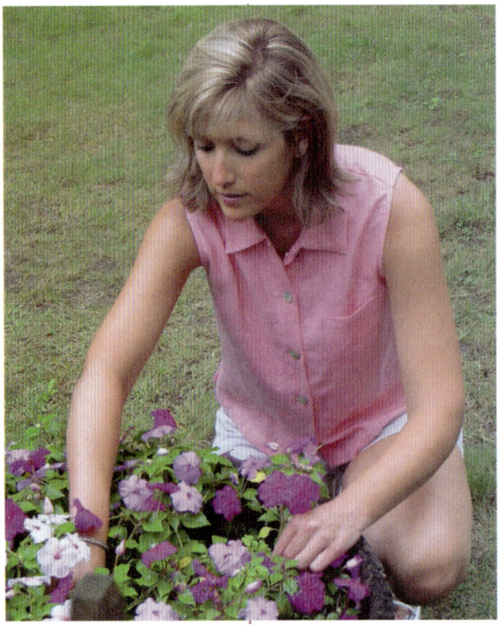

If your goal is to climb the stairs unaided, you *can* make it to the top, slowly but surely. Or if you have trouble rising from a chair after sitting down, you *can* achieve a painless liftoff. It's a matter of assessing your problem, setting reasonable goals, and then working to achieve those goals. You will be able to measure your progress in the form of reduced pain, greater mobility, and enhanced well-being.

The Eight Steps for Overcoming Arthritis

This self-help approach has already liberated thousands of arthritis patients from a life of pain and disability. Why? Because at the core of the plan is an incontrovertible premise: No one cares about your welfare as much as you do. Not your doctor, family, or friends.

As many patients have found out, thoroughly educating yourself about your condition and the treatments available is a giant step toward that liberation. Just because you have a chronic disease doesn't mean it has to rule your life. Digesting and incorporating these eight steps into your daily life will empower you to gain the upper hand over your arthritis.

1 Get to know your problem

The more you know about a problem, the better you'll be able to deal with it. And the better acquainted you are with arthritis, the better equipped you'll be to overcome it. This isn't a very profound insight, but it is a very powerful one. In *Taking Charge of Arthritis*, you'll learn the answers to vitally important questions about your particular type of arthritis, such as "What causes it?" "How is it diagnosed?" "What are the best treatments available?"

This insightful book will help you analyze your individual problem: Is pain the most troublesome symptom you have? If so, how bad is it? Is it worse in the morning or later in the day? By answering these and other questions, you'll be able to develop an effective anti-arthritis program tailored to your needs.

2 Choose your long-term goal

Chances are you want to resume a much-loved activity—going for a walk on the beach or playing with the children or grandchildren, for example—that arthritis has taken away from you. The best goals are specific, well-defined ones such as "I want to be able to walk a mile without knee pain." It's easier to motivate yourself to achieve a specific goal than a vague goal and also easier to tell whether you have attained it. Whatever it is, carving out a clear-cut goal can provide the motivation you need to jump-start your arthritis self-management plan.

3 Decide on a strategy

Once you have your goal, you need a treatment strategy for reaching it. Certainly, there are no lack of treatment approaches available. Books, websites, news segments on the latest arthritis treatments—patients have a confusing glut of information to contend with. Do you want to eliminate the pain in your arthritic knee? If so, you could take a number of approaches including weight loss, an exercise program, or using anti-inflammatory drugs. Do you want to take a load off your knees by losing 20 pounds? You could skip high-calorie desserts, begin an exercise program, decrease your portion sizes, or take your lunch to work instead of eating out. Or you could combine several of these approaches into your overall strategy.

what the studies show

Arthritis patients who actively participate in their own care report less pain, require fewer doctor visits, and enjoy a better quality of life. In one recent study of participants in an arthritis self-help program, patients who completed the program reported nearly a 20 percent reduction in pain and 40 percent fewer doctor visits than nonparticipants. And the benefits of participating in the program lasted for four years.

The Many Faces of Arthritis

Arthritis is not a single disease but actually encompasses a total of 127 separate disorders. They include ones you're probably familiar with such as osteoarthritis, rheumatoid arthritis and gout, and much rarer types such as psoriatic arthritis (see Chapter 2). Although many of these 100-plus disorders have very different causes and symptoms, they do share a common feature: All of them involve inflammation of the joints. Indeed, the term "arthritis" comes from the Greek words *arthron* (which means joint) and *itis* (which means inflammation).

No goal worth achieving can be reached overnight or without effort. An effective anti-arthritis strategy will require some work or even some sacrifices (forgoing those tasty desserts, for example), but reaching your goal will ultimately make it all worthwhile.

4 Draw up your weekly take-charge plan

For someone with arthritis, that old Chinese saying, "A journey of a thousand miles must begin with a single step," is literally and figuratively true. In creating your weekly take-charge plan you decide on a short-term goal and then assign yourself specific actions for achieving that goal.

A positive attitude is even more important to a patient's success than following her doctor's advice on treatment, nutrition, or exercise.

If you want to lose 20 pounds, for example, your weekly take-charge plan might call for a short-term goal of losing one pound. Then you get down to specific weight loss actions, eliminating fatty desserts, for example, or walking to burn up calories. If you complete those actions with relatively little effort, you can write in slightly more ambitious actions for next week's plan.

Build a team. It's wise to be inclusive when drawing up your take-charge plan. Solicit input from your doctor, especially if you haven't yet been diagnosed with arthritis or don't know what kind you have. Many people assume that their aches and pains stem from arthritis, but sometimes their problems are caused by something else entirely, such as an adverse reaction to a drug, an infection, or even a malignancy. So if you're not sure whether you have arthritis, now is the time to see your doctor before trying to manage a condition you might not even have!

If you have been diagnosed with arthritis, work closely with your doctor to draw up a take-charge plan and put it into action. See you and your doctor as a team, and see yourself as the quarterback. A good partnership with your doctor can greatly assist you in achieving your goals. In Chapter 4, *Working with Your Doctor*, we will tell you how to get the most out of this relationship, with advice on choosing a doctor if you need one, preparing for office visits, asking the right questions once you go, and building a strong team of players—from family to a physical therapist to possibly an acupuncturist.

5 Put your take-charge plan into action

Now comes the hard part: following through on the strategy you've devised. If your goal of losing a pound over the next week calls for cutting out 500 calories per day, you may have to skip that morning doughnut and afternoon cappuccino.

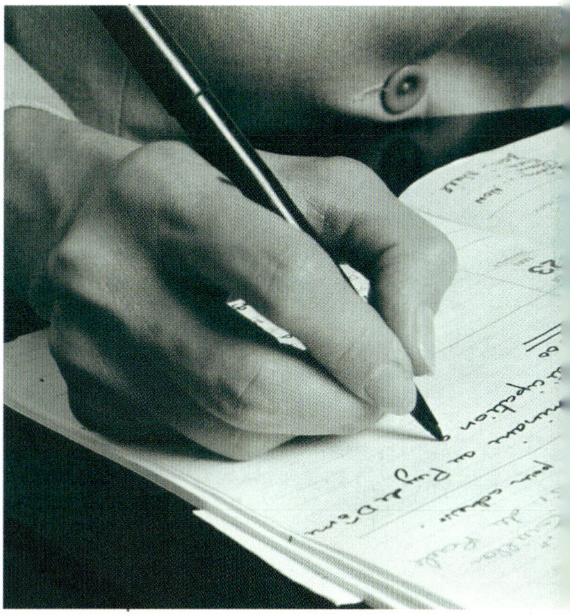

6 Monitor your progress

As the week passes, note how well you've done in completing the actions you've assigned yourself in your take-charge plan. Congratulate yourself if you've been able to stick to your plan, but don't punish or berate yourself if you did some backsliding. Nobody ever said that changing a habit was easy.

7 Adjust your action plan

If you don't attain the short-term goal called for in your weekly take-charge plan, figure out what went wrong and identify a way to correct it. If you lost only half a pound, maybe losing one pound a week was too ambitious. Or, as it turned out, maybe one pound was easy and you could safely lose a little more. Either way, you probably need to fine-tune your action plan.

8 Build on your success

Success, as we know, is one of the best of all motivators. If you've achieved your short-term goal for one week, the momentum from that success will carry over into the following week—and inspire you to set a more ambitious goal. As you target and attain new goals, you'll find yourself actually overcoming your arthritis in the process.

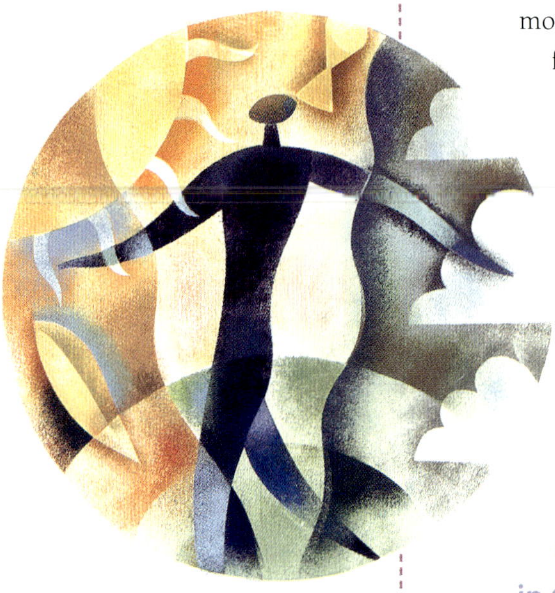

The Secrets of Self-Treatment

In drawing up your self-management plan, you'll probably incorporate a smorgasbord of therapies. As you do so, keep in mind that people vary widely in their responses to therapies. This is called bio-individuality.

Very simply, it means that individuals with similar symptoms will respond differently to the same treatment. What helps your arthritis pain might not help your brother-in-law's. So be patient and open-minded as you tick off and try out therapies for your condition.

now and then

As recently as 20 years ago, doctors advised arthritis patients against exercising for fear that it would worsen joint damage and inflammation. But it's now recognized that moderate physical activity can be one of the most effective of all arthritis treatments.

BONING UP: Surgery to repair or replace arthritic joints is a last resort—but can produce dramatic results. For example, surgical procedures for implanting artificial hips and knees have greatly improved in recent years and can virtually eliminate pain and disability due to arthritis.

Help yourself. As you'll learn in this book, some of the most effective anti-arthritis therapies don't involve drugs, but instead are things you can do for yourself every day. Unfortunately, many

caution

If you take vitamin E, formulations containing gamma tocopherol may actually make arthritis worse. Researchers at the University of North Carolina measured blood levels of two forms of vitamin E (gamma tocopherol and alpha tocopherol) in 400 volunteers. X rays revealed that the volunteers with high blood levels of gamma tocopherol were much more likely to have developed osteoarthritis. So avoid brands of vitamin E labeled as "E-complex" or "mixed tocopherols," the ones most likely to contain gamma tocopherol. Instead look for ones with only alpha tocopherol.

doctors fail to recommend nondrug therapies for their arthritis patients—despite considerable evidence that such therapies can be quite effective in relieving pain and disability. *Taking Charge of Arthritis* gives you a practical plan for using nutrition, exercise, dietary supplements, and other do-it-yourself therapies to treat your arthritis. For example, in these pages you'll find invaluable strategies and techniques to:

Lose weight

Losing just a few pounds can relieve your knee pain as effectively as the most potent painkiller. If your goal is to lose weight, you'll learn about tried-and-true weight-loss strategies that will help you lose the pounds and keep them off.

Take the right vitamins

The Framingham Osteoarthritis Study (part of the long-running Framingham Heart Study) has found that diets rich in certain vitamins may slow down the progression of osteoarthritis or even prevent the disease from occurring. *Taking Charge of Arthritis* gives you the inside scoop on the vitamins that can make a big difference in your condition, along with how much of each you should take.

Exercise pain away

Studies during the past decade have shown that strengthening the muscles that surround and support the joints can yield valuable payoffs in the form of reduced pain and greater mobility. For example, strengthening your thigh muscles can dramatically relieve pain and stiffness in osteoarthritis of the knees. You'll learn

what the studies show

In a new and surprising study, people with rheumatoid arthritis who simply wrote about stressful events in their lives experienced significant reductions in their symptoms.

about these simple exercises as well as many others, including such exotic but effective therapies as yoga and tai chi.

De-stress yourself

Stress doesn't cause arthritis, but there is ample evidence that stress can worsen the condition—especially by increasing the muscle tension that can aggravate joint pain. *Taking Charge of Arthritis* clues you into the best techniques for defusing the stress in your life, including mind-body approaches that can do so much to help arthritis patients.

Take an alternative approach

Three dietary supplements have shown genuine value in treating arthritis...while other highly touted treatments waste your time and money and could jeopardize your health. *Taking Charge of Arthritis* takes a hard look at the science behind "alternative" therapies and concludes which can help you and which can harm you.

did you know

Smoking cigarettes can worsen the symptoms of rheumatoid arthritis and is considered to be a risk factor in triggering the disease. Smoking may cause abnormalities in the immune system of rheumatoid arthritis patients.

Saying Yes to Drugs

Self-help measures may be all you need to control and overcome your arthritis, and you won't need to rely on the arsenal of arthritis drugs.

But for many people, prescription and over-the-counter drugs remain crucially important for treating their condition. In the past few years, researchers have made great strides in developing safer and better medications to battle the pain of arthritis, some of which you may not have heard about. Here's a sampling of the cutting-edge treatments you'll learn about in this book:

- **Severe rheumatoid arthritis** doesn't need to be a crippling disorder. A new class of drugs, called the disease-modifying anti-rheumatic drugs (DMARDs), has revolutionized the treatment of the highly painful, disfiguring condition. Recent studies show that these drugs may actually slow or even halt the joint damage that occurs in rheumatoid arthritis. The availability of these drugs should mean that many fewer patients will be crippled by their disease.
- **Three recently approved** nonsteroidal anti-inflammatory drugs—Celebrex, Mobic, and Vioxx—can relieve arthritis

pain and inflammation as effectively as traditional NSAIDs while posing much less risk of potentially fatal side effects such as stomach bleeding. And although some standard NSAIDs may damage cartilage when used regularly—something even many doctors don't know about!—these three new drugs probably don't pose that risk.

- **Two revolutionary liquids**—Synvisc and Hyalan—can be injected directly into the knee joint weekly for three to five weeks to lubricate and nourish cartilage. Both of these recently approved substances are derived from the combs of roosters and contain hyaluronic acid, a normal component of the joint's synovial fluid. According to recent studies, these products can relieve pain for months and may be ideal for people with osteoarthritis of the knee who've failed to respond to or couldn't tolerate other forms of treatment.

In addition, *Taking Charge of Arthritis* will also tell you about a wide range of promising treatments—from antibiotic therapy to gene therapy—now being investigated that may be available to you soon.

on the horizon

In 1990, a study in the *New England Journal of Medicine* reported that osteoarthritis can be caused by an inherited genetic abnormality. Experts now believe that at least 25 percent of all cases of osteoarthritis have a genetic basis. Several teams of researchers are now working to develop gene therapy for the condition.

An Ancient Disorder

If you think arthritis is mostly a modern-day affliction, you would be wrong: It is one of the oldest ailments known to man and beast.

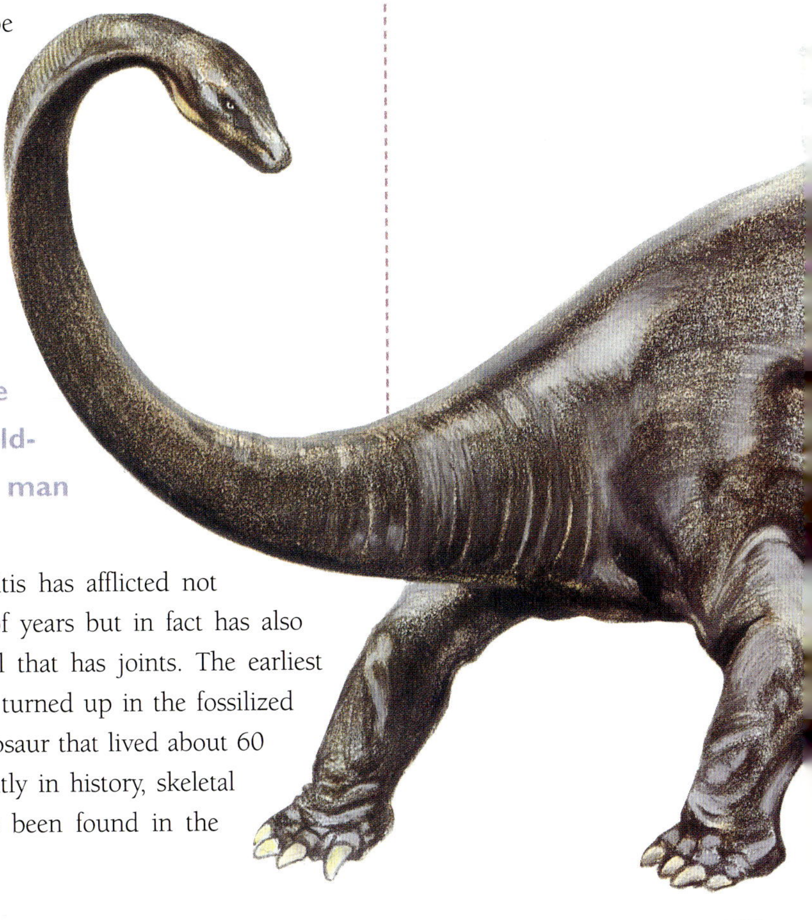

Evidence shows that arthritis has afflicted not only humans for thousands of years but in fact has also affected virtually every animal that has joints. The earliest known signs of arthritis have turned up in the fossilized skeleton of Diplodocus, a dinosaur that lived about 60 million years ago. More recently in history, skeletal evidence of osteoarthritis has been found in the remains of Neanderthal man and in Egyptian mummies. In fact, a 5,300-year-old mummy, nicknamed Oetzi, is believed to have suffered from arthritis, and the numerous tattoos on his body may have been an ancient therapy for his condition.

Through the centuries, arthritis has obviously been an important and widespread human affliction. Artists have long used bent-backed human figures and hands with gnarled fingers to symbolize the frailty of old age. Shakespeare referred to arthritic diseases in *A Midsummer Night's Dream* ("Therefore the moon.../Pale in her anger, washes all the air/ That rheumatic diseases do abound"), and John Milton cited them in *Paradise Lost*: "Disease is a consequence of man's imperfection—dropsies, asthmas, and joint-wracking rheumatism."

did you know

Arthritis costs the U.S. economy nearly $65 billion annually in medical expenses and lost wages—an impact equal to a moderate recession.

From Caveman to Modern Man

Arthritis remains a widespread affliction today. It is the most common of all chronic diseases, affecting more Americans than heart disease, cancer, or diabetes.

According to the latest estimates from the U.S. Centers for Disease Control and Prevention, some 43 million Americans now have arthritis—which means one in every seven Americans and one third of all families are affected.

The cost of arthritis. Osteoarthritis accounts for more than seven million visits to doctors each year due to pain and limited mobility, as well as 36 million lost workdays. Arthritis patients make 7.8 visits to the physician annually—more than twice as many as those without the condition. These figures

Arthritis Through the Ages

30,000 B.C. — Neanderthal man emerges, and his fossilized remains reveal many cases of osteoarthritis resulting from injuries.

3,000 B.C. — "The Iceman" dies while hiking in the Alps on the present-day Austria-Italian border. Examination of his frozen corpse reveals that he had arthritic joints.

4th century B.C. — 18 of Hippocrates' aphorisms referred to joint ailments, five of them pertaining to gout.

44 B.C. — Famous Romans Julius Caesar (died 44 B.C.) and Horace (satirist, born 65 B.C.) both had arthritis.

300 A.D. — Roman Emperor Diocletian exempts citizens with severe arthritis from taxation.

Ailments by the Numbers

Here are the leading causes of disability among persons aged 15 years or older in the United States.

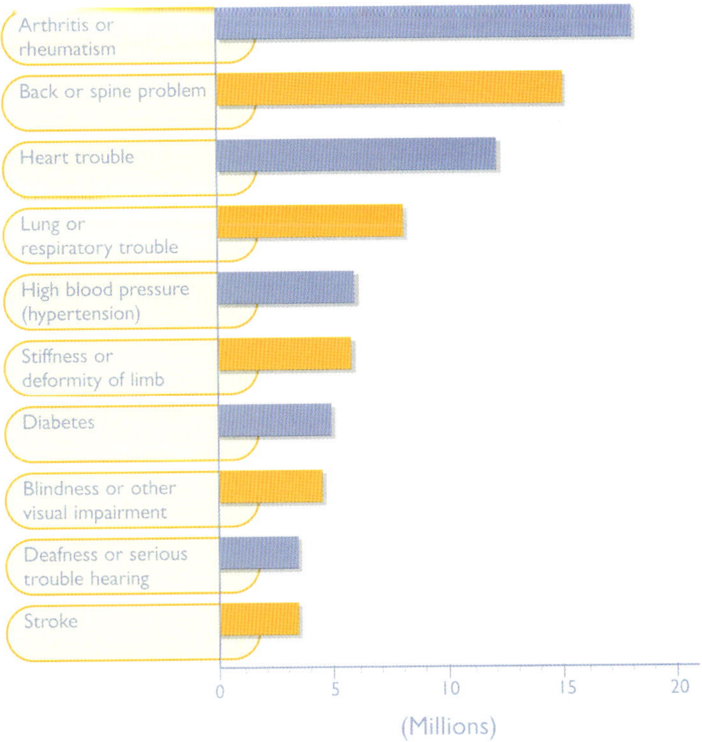

will only increase in the coming years: According to federal estimates, arthritis cases will rise dramatically as Baby Boomers begin approaching retirement age, surging to 60 million by the year 2020.

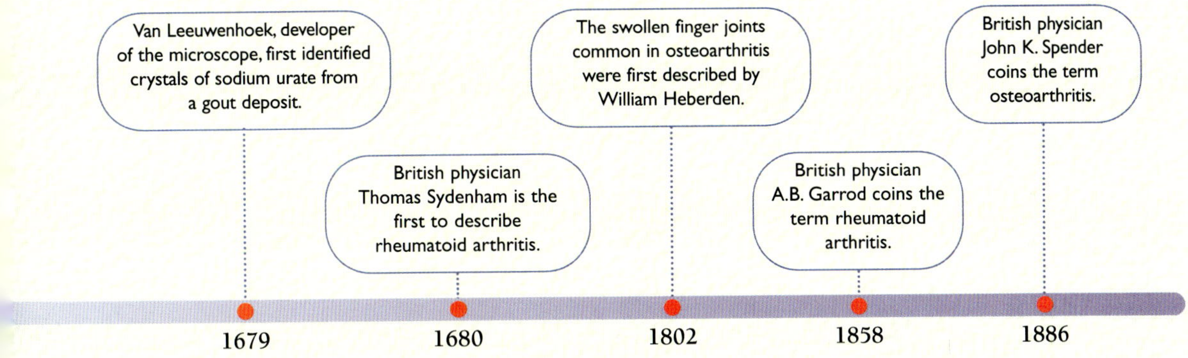

Survey Says?

Adults with arthritis are substantially worse off than others when it comes to health-related quality of life, according to a report from the U.S. Centers for Disease Control and Prevention. Researchers surveyed more than 32,000 Americans in 11 states, 29 percent of whom reported having arthritis. "Respondents with arthritis reported having fair or poor health approximately three times more often than respondents without arthritis," the researchers wrote.

Behind the numbers is the physical toll that arthritis exacts. Arthritis is the nation's leading cause of disability: More than seven million Americans with arthritis have trouble performing everyday activities such as getting dressed, climbing stairs, or getting in and out of bed. In addition, arthritis is the main cause of limited mobility in the elderly.

As grim as these statistics seem, there has been exciting progress on the research front in targeting the causes of the condition. Osteoarthritis, by far the most common form of arthritis, was once considered a normal and inevitable part of aging. But researchers have recently uncovered a number of causes for osteoarthritis, some of which—such as obesity and injuries to the joint—can be corrected in time to prevent the disease.

1896 — The first X ray of joints affected by rheumatoid arthritis is published.

1897 — German chemist Felix Hoffman synthesizes aspirin while searching for a treatment for his father's arthritis.

1933 — Swedish ophthalmologist Henrik Sjögren describes the condition that will be named in his honor as Sjögren's syndrome.

1955 — Tylenol, the world's leading acetaminophen product, is introduced as an aspirin-free pain reliever.

1977 — The genetic marker HLA-DR4 is found to be associated with rheumatoid arthritis.

BONING UP: Contrary to what many of us have heard, cracking your knuckles doesn't lead to arthritis. The cracking sound is simply caused by a rapid release of synovial fluid inside the joint, not by any damage to the joint. Although the sound may be unpleasant, the act is harmless.

Exploring estrogen. Women suffer from osteoarthritis more than men, comprising three quarters of all cases in the US. Some researchers have theorized that this correlation is due to the diminishing levels of the female sex hormone, estrogen, as women age. Scientists already know that lower levels of the hormone at menopause leads to brittle bones and are exploring the relationship between estrogen and osteoarthritis. Researchers found that women who received supplemental estrogen for 10 years or longer had a greater reduction in the risk of any hip osteoarthritis as compared to those who took it for less than 10 years. More research is needed, but certainly the estrogen connection may lead to less suffering in women in the future.

Researchers aren't just dwelling on the causes of osteoarthritis; they are exploring new avenues of treatment for people already suffering with long-term aches and pain. Acupuncture, the ancient treatment that has been used to relieve painful conditions

1981 Swiss biologist Willy Burgdorfer, working in the U.S., discovers that Lyme disease, a trigger for rheumatoid arthritis, is caused by a microorganism that is transmitted by tick bites.

1988 The FDA approves the cancer drug methotrexate for treating rheumatoid arthritis.

1990 Scientists discover the first genetic defect involved in causing osteoarthritis in some families.

1998 The FDA approves Celebrex, the first COX-2 inhibitor, a new class of nonsteroidal anti-inflammatory drugs that causes less stomach upset than traditional NSAIDs.

1999 Experts predict that the number of Americans with arthritis will increase sharply, from 43 million to nearly 60 million in 2020.

for thousands of years, might be potent against osteoarthritis of the knee. A study reported in 1997 by the University of Maryland suggests that the therapy, especially when combined with conventional medical therapy, reduces pain in an osteoarthritic knee.

> "I don't think many people realize how large a problem (arthritis) is. These are big numbers that are going to get a lot bigger."
>
> —Chad Helmick, M.D.

New insights about rheumatoid arthritis. Rheumatoid arthritis is also revealing its secrets to researchers, who have found that a naturally occurring protein—tumor necrosis factor—plays a crucial role in causing joint inflammation and damage. Through genetic engineering, researchers have developed two new drugs, Enbrel and Remicade, that block tumor necrosis factor. These and other new "disease-modifying" drugs have revolutionized the way rheumatoid arthritis is treated.

Much talked about these days is minocycline, an antibiotic from the tetracycline family that was originally used to treat acne. The medication may block enzymes that destroy cartilage inside joints. In addition, a very promising treatment that may actually cure rheumatoid arthritis was reported late last year. Developed by researchers at University College in London, the new treatment involves depleting the blood of B lymphocytes; these immune cells form antibodies that cause much of the joint destruction that occurs in rheumatoid arthritis.

on the horizon

The National Institutes of Health's National Center for Complementary and Alternative Medicine has begun two clinical trials for the treatment of osteoarthritis. One will test glucosamine and chondroitin sulfate, two of the most promising dietary supplements for treating osteoarthritis. The second trial will evaluate acupuncture for the treatment of pain associated with osteoarthritis. Results from both trials should be available by 2002.

Attacking Arthritis: A National Game Plan

Researchers aren't the only ones trying to get to the bottom of the condition. The national rise of arthritis has clearly galvanized the efforts of the country's public health officials.

In 1999, three national organizations—the Arthritis Foundation, the Centers for Disease Control and Prevention, and the Association of State and Territorial Health Officials—joined forces to attack the public health challenges posed by arthritis. Their effort, known as The National Arthritis Action Plan: A Public Health Strategy, has six goals:

- Increase public awareness of arthritis as the leading cause of disability and an important health problem
- Prevent arthritis whenever possible

Exorcising Pain Before Exercise

There are known methods of stopping arthritis pain for short periods of time. Here are several methods you can use before exercising or just going to the grocery store:

Moist heat: Warm towels, hot packs, a bath, or a shower can relieve pain when done 15 to 20 minutes three times a day.

Cold: A bag of ice wrapped in a towel helps to stop pain and reduce swelling when used for 10 to 15 minutes at a time. This is especially effective for inflamed joints.

Relaxation therapy: Patients can learn to release the tension in their muscles to relieve pain.

Mobilization therapies: Traction (gentle, steady pulling), massage, and manipulation (using the hands to restore normal movement to stiff joints) can all help control pain and increase joint motion and muscle and tendon flexibility.

- Promote early diagnosis and appropriate management for people with arthritis to ensure they have as many years of healthy life as they can
- Minimize preventable pain and disability due to arthritis
- Support people with arthritis in developing and accessing the resources they need to cope with their disease
- Ensure that people with arthritis receive the family, peer, and community support they need

As you can see, the war on arthritis is a full-fledged effort. But until more progress is made, you will continue to be the architect of how you live with it. You will need to take those first proactive steps that will help you lead as normal a life as possible. And you can do it with *Taking Charge of Arthritis* by your side. The book gives you everything you need for achieving your goals: guidance in becoming a self-manager of your arthritis and the latest information on the pain-relieving treatments that best fit your needs.

did you know

Switching from high heels to flats may decrease a woman's chances of developing osteoarthritis. One study done in England claims that women who walk in high-heeled shoes strain the area between the kneecap and the thighbone, especially in the inner side of the joint. This joint strain may contribute to osteoarthritis.

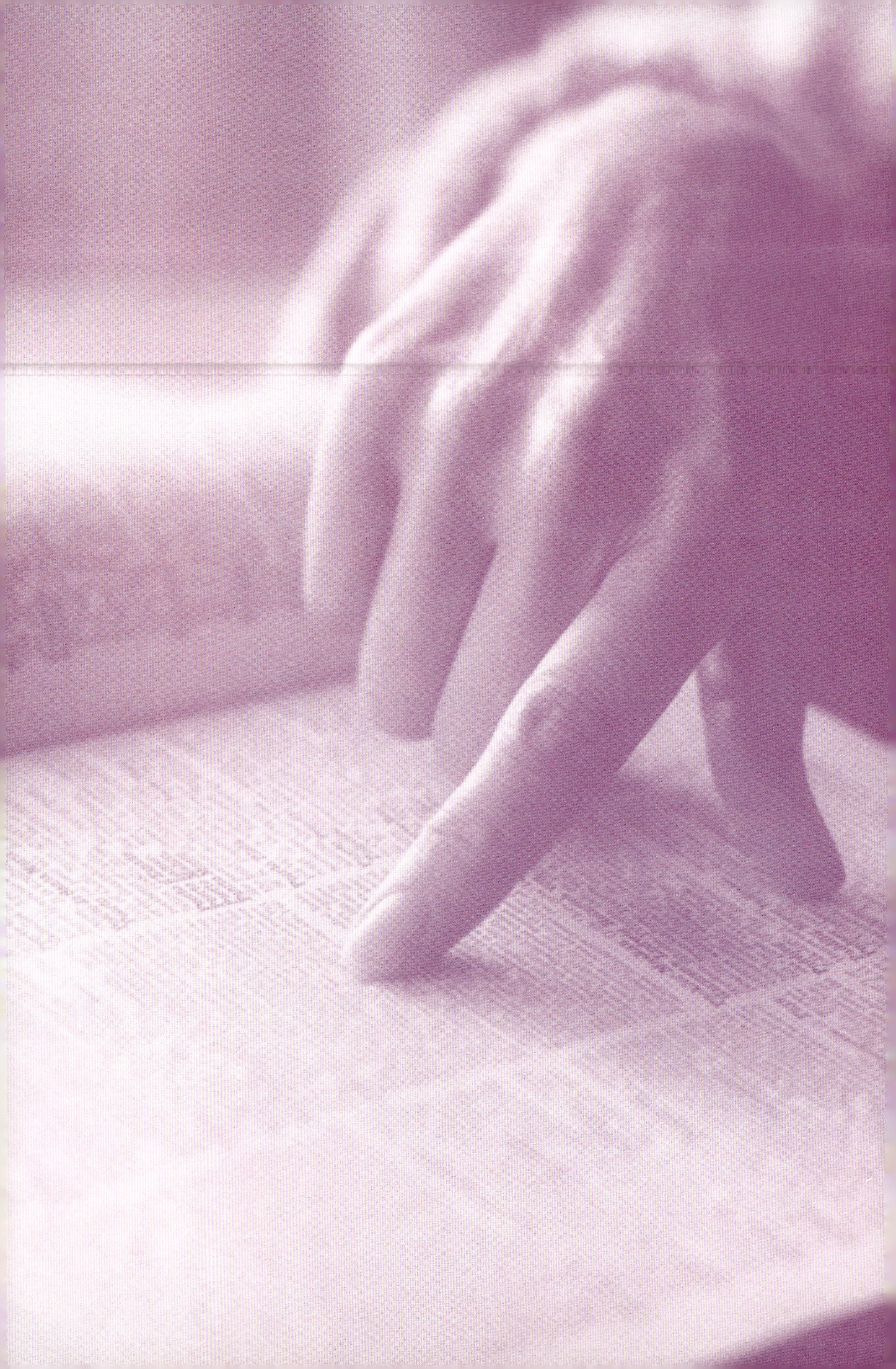

2 Know Your Arthritis

Knowing how a healthy body works and
then understanding what goes wrong
when arthritis attacks can help you get
the upper hand on treatment and pain relief.
It will also transform you into a motivated,
full-time partner in your own health care.

KEY CONCEPT

The more you know about your particular type of arthritis, the greater your chances of overcoming the pain and the limitations it imposes on you.

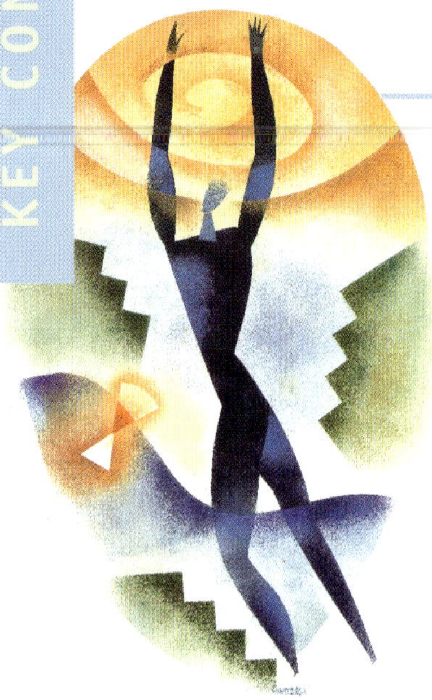

Knowledge Is Power

Many people suffering with arthritis are caught up in a devastating cycle of pain, depression, and stress. Becoming an active participant in managing your pain, however, can break that vicious cycle. Boning up on your condition also takes personal fear out of the arthritis equation. Knowing what's going on with your body can impose a much-needed sense of calm and enable you to make clear-headed decisions.

An Equal-Opportunity Condition

Arthritis should always be referred to in the plural sense because it encompasses some 127 different diseases. So when you say, "I have arthritis," the logical response is, "What kind?" Arthritis, in its many forms, can strike all ages and both sexes. Some forms—rheumatoid arthritis, fibromyalgia, and lupus—are more prevalent among women; gout and ankylosing spondylitis are more common in men.

Indeed, arthritis has many faces. It may affect only one joint or it may involve an immune attack against many of them. You may experience only mild pain while someone else may suffer from excruciating aches and extreme fatigue. Your symptoms may fluctuate between great pain and periods of quiescence while a friend's symptoms may remain stable for years. Some forms of the disease are caused by metabolic disorders, others are due to genes (congenital defects in the joints), and still others may result from environmental factors—what we do or don't eat, for example.

Arthritis primer. This chapter will thoroughly ground you

The Feminine Side of Arthritis

According to the Arthritis Foundation, some 26 million women of all ages suffer from some type of arthritis—nearly two thirds of all Americans living with the disease. Theories abound, including women's weaker cartilage and tendons, and a possible link to the female sex hormone, estrogen. All remain unproven, but one thing is for sure: the statistical evidence underscoring women's affliction with the condition. For example:

Osteoarthritis affects 15.3 million women (representing 74 percent of all cases).

Rheumatoid arthritis affects 1.5 million women (representing 71 percent of all cases).

Systemic lupus erythematosus (SLE) affects 117,000 women (representing 90 percent of all cases).

Fibromyalgia affects an estimated 3.7 million Americans, mostly women.

Juvenile rheumatoid arthritis affects up to 50,000 children (with girls representing 86 percent of all cases).

in the most common types of arthritis. In each case, we describe the condition and explain its causes and the progression of symptoms. We also provide you with an invaluable rundown about how each type of arthritis should be diagnosed, what you should do once you are diagnosed, and, of course, the most promising treatments. In later chapters, we'll tell you much more about treatments—the exercises, drugs, nutrition, stress-reduction techniques, and alternative approaches that can help you overcome your arthritis problem. We begin with a primer on the anatomy of a joint—ground zero for virtually every type of arthritis.

Bones and Joints 101

Bones are connected to each other at joints. The body's joints can be grouped into three classes based on the amount of movement they allow: fixed joints, slightly movable joints, and freely movable joints.

Fixed joints. These joints allow no movement whatever. Examples of fixed joints include those separating the bones of the pelvis, which bend only during delivery to ease the baby's movement down the birth canal, and the joints (known as sutures) between the bones of the skull.

Slightly movable joints. These joints allow a limited amount of motion. For example, the bones of the spinal column are held together by tough pads (or "disks") of fibrocartilage. These so-called intervertebral joints secure the bones tightly, but do provide some flexibility, allowing you to bend and stretch.

Freely movable joints. Also known as synovial joints, they usually leap to mind when we think of arthritis. Examples are

Name That Joint

You know them by the names elbow, shoulder, and knee. But every joint in the body also has a scientific name as well. Take this little anatomical quiz, trying to match each of the numbered joints on the left with its scientific moniker on the right.

1. Shoulder
2. Knee
3. Wrist
4. Joint that connects a spinal vertebra
5. Joint where spine joins pelvis
6. Joint where ribs join breastbone
7. Finger joint
8. Joint at the base of the thumb
9. Bunion joint at the base of the toe

- A. Sacroiliac
- B. Costochondral joint
- C. First metatarsophalangeal joint
- D. Glenohumeral
- E. Tibiofemoral
- F. Radiocarpal
- G. Facet joint
- H. Interphalangeal joint
- I. First carpometacarpal joint

Answers: 1) D; 2) E; 3) F; 4) G; 5) A; 6) B; 7) H; 8) I; 9) C the hips, knees, elbows, fingers and—most mobile of all—the shoulder joint, whose ball-and-socket structure enables you to move your arm in a complete circle.

BONING UP: The human skeleton contains more than 200 bones, which are connected by almost 150 joints.

did you know

By age 65, more than half of all people have x-ray evidence of osteoarthritis in at least one joint.

Joints: How Things Work

The freely movable joints are the prime location for many types of arthritis, including the two most common—osteoarthritis and rheumatoid arthritis. Chances are that your arthritis affects one or more of your synovial joints, so you need to know your way around them and have an idea of the key players involved in their everyday operation.

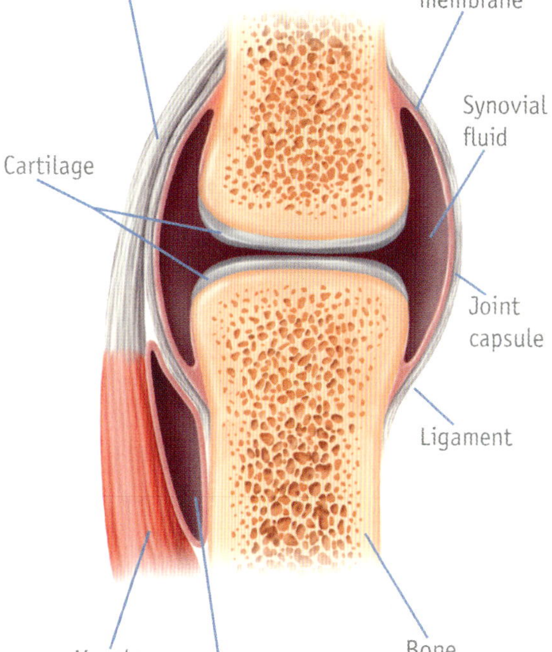

Bones

The ends of bones form the heart of a synovial joint. When you bend, twist, or turn, joints provide the flexibility to move these bones into position. Most of our everyday actions—walking, sitting down, washing dishes—require the smooth movement of bones within the joints.

Articular cartilage

This is a rubbery, gel-like tissue that sits at the end of the bones where they meet at a joint. Cartilage provides a smooth surface so that bones can move easily through their range of motion without grating against each other. This smooth movement is aided by the slippery synovial fluid that bathes the joint. Articular (which simply means joint) cartilage also plays a crucial shock-absorbing role.

When you run, for instance, you exert between four and eight times your body's weight on your knees and hips. Even ordinary walking can double the weight on those joints with every step

Bursitis: Cushions in Crisis

Small sacs called bursae are found near certain joints, including the elbow and knee. They're filled with synovial fluid and act as cushions, taking the pressure off the surface of a bone or easing the friction created on tendons or muscles when a joint is in motion.

Bursitis—inflammation of one or more bursae—usually occurs when people repeatedly put pressure on a joint. For example, students who prop their heads on their elbows while studying may develop "student's elbow." Or carpet installers, who must kneel for long periods of time, may develop bursitis of the knee.

Bursitis or arthritis? Bursitis is a "local" problem—only the bursae are affected—but is often mistaken for arthritis. The inflammation causes pain, tenderness, and sometimes swelling; moving the joint often makes the problem worse. Anti-inflammatory drugs such as aspirin or ibuprofen can sometimes help, and so can applying an ice pack. But often the best treatment for bursitis is simply to rest the affected joint, which allows the excess fluid inside the bursa to become reabsorbed into the bloodstream.

you take. Exercise can stimulate the healthy flow of synovial fluid into and out of the cartilage. When there is no pressure on a joint, synovial fluid flows into the cartilage, bathing it in nutrients needed to strengthen the tissue and maintain its health. When pressure is exerted—when you run or walk, for example—the fluid seeps out of the cartilage, absorbing and dispersing the pressure. Without synovial fluid pulsing through it regularly, cartilage would slowly dry out.

BONING UP: Every extra pound of weight you put on adds four to eight pounds more stress on the knees and hips.

Joint capsule

The bones of the joint are covered by a tough, fibrous covering called the joint capsule. The capsule's outer layer is made of interwoven bands of collagen fibers that provide the joint capsule with strength and flexibility.

Synovial membrane

The joint capsule's inner surface is lined with a delicate layer of tissue called the synovial membrane, which contains cells that produce and release synovial fluid. This clear, yellow, sticky fluid is 95 percent water, has the consistency of egg white (*synovia* means "like egg white"), and helps nourish and lubricate the cartilage and bones within the joint capsule. Aided by the synovial fluid, the cartilage-tipped bones in a healthy joint glide over each other smoothly, creating even less friction than ice sliding on ice.

Ligaments

These strong, flexible bands of tissue help to stabilize the joint by binding together the bones within it. Most ligaments lack elasticity, but some do stretch to allow slight separation of the bones that they connect.

Tendons

Also known as sinews, they assist the ligaments in stabilizing and supporting the joints. These strong white cords of fibrous tissue serve to attach muscles to the bones of the joint.

Muscles

They provide the forces that move the bones within a joint. Even the simplest movement requires at least two muscles acting in equal and opposite ways: One contracts and pulls on its attached tendon, which in turn pulls on a bone and moves it. At the same time, the opposing muscle relaxes to allow the movement to occur.

what the studies show

Exercises that protect and strengthen the muscles, tendons, and ligaments that surround a joint can minimize pain and stiffness within the joint itself.

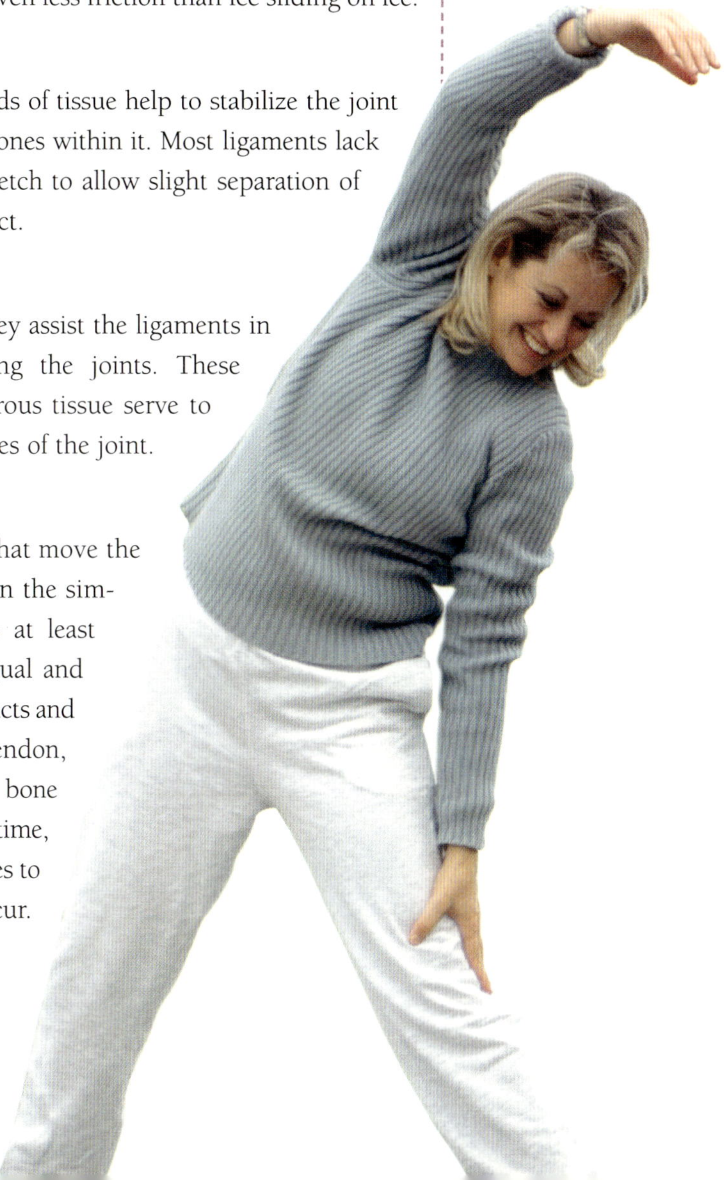

did you know

- Osteoarthritis has been found in all mammals except those, including bats and sloths, that spend most of their lives hanging upside down.
- The National Institutes of Health spent $3.4 billion on cancer research in 1999, but only $237 million on arthritis research.

Osteoarthritis: Good Cartilage Gone Bad

Osteoarthritis (OA) is by far the most common type of arthritis, affecting some 21 million Americans, about half of all Americans who have some form of arthritis. Many people call it "old folks' arthritis" or degenerative joint disease, but it can happen to younger folks, too. Whatever your age, OA needs to be approached with an informed strategy.

What Is OA?

Since *osteo* is the Greek word for bone, you may have thought that osteoarthritis is a bone disorder. But actually the condition mainly involves cartilage, the protective tissue that covers and cushions the ends of the bones within the joint.

Boning Up: Osteoarthritis can occur in any joint in the body, but most commonly affects the hips, knees, lower back, neck, and fingers. OA in the wrists, elbows, and ankles can often be traced to an injury or to a job that subjects them to repeated stress.

Dysfunctional cartilage. In OA, the cartilage doesn't function as it was intended and, for a variety of reasons, slowly breaks down. A number of possible causes—injury to the cartilage, genetic mutations, factors associated with aging—precipitate the breakdown. The result? The cartilage wears away—which is why osteoarthritis is sometimes referred to as "wear-and-tear" or "degenerative" arthritis. As the cartilage erodes, joints no longer move smoothly but instead feel—and sometimes sound—creaky.

Most OA sufferers have what is called primary OA, meaning the cause of their cartilage breakdown isn't known. In cases of secondary OA, cartilage damage can be traced to a specific cause such as a physical injury to the joint, inflammation due to rheumatoid arthritis, or misaligned bones.

Unlike some other types of arthritis—rheumatoid arthritis, for instance—OA affects only the joints and not any other parts of the body. Not surprisingly, OA is most likely to develop in those joints that are subject to the greatest amount of stress: the body's weight-bearing joints, especially the knees and hips.

Cartilage: The Inside Story

Water

Articular cartilage is mostly water—80 percent, in fact. Its high water content helps cartilage cushion the bones from trauma. Cartilage derives its water from the synovial fluid that bathes and lubricates the bones in a joint.

Collagen

This protein comes in the form of rod-shaped fibers that are the main building block for skin, tendons, bones, and other connective tissues. As a key ingredient in cartilage, collagen strengthens cartilage and helps it resist being pulled apart by pressure or other traumas.

Proteoglycans

Cartilage owes its high water content to proteoglycans—molecules that have the unique ability to soak up and hold fluid in the cartilage, allowing it to flow in and out as the pressure on a joint increases and decreases. Strands of proteoglycans team up with collagen to form a weblike, water-filled matrix that provides cartilage with its sponge-like resilience, its ability to absorb pressure, and its surface slickness. OA begins with the breakdown of this matrix of proteoglycans and collagen.

Chondrocytes

Scattered throughout cartilage, these cartilage-producing cells are responsible for synthesizing and repairing the cartilage "scaffolding"—namely, its collagen and proteoglycan molecules.

The road to osteoarthritis. As cartilage breaks down, it can no longer cushion bones or prevent bones from rubbing against each other. In addition, bony swellings or spurs (known as osteophytes) may develop around the edge of bones in response to pressure on them. These changes lead to the symptoms that people with OA know all too well: pain, stiffness, and restricted range of motion.

What Causes OA?

The cause of primary osteoarthritis—what triggers joint cartilage to erode—is not yet known. The disease process apparently begins when destructive enzymes damage the network of collagen fibers

Debunking Cartilage Myths

Until recently, osteoarthritis was wrongly viewed as a natural consequence of getting older—an inevitable result of decades of wear and tear on the joints. But scientists studying cartilage have made some exciting discoveries suggesting that the cartilage breakdown leading to osteoarthritis is by no means inevitable.

It's alive. Once considered simple and inert, cartilage is living tissue. A hotbed of metabolic activity, cartilage is constantly being both produced and broken down. In fact, a dietary supplement, chondroitin sulfate, may help rebuild cartilage by suppressing enzymes that destroy cartilage. Drugs that may achieve the same result are now being studied.

The right stuff. In an important study, researchers analyzed joint cartilage from elderly people with osteoarthritis and from people the same age who were free of the disease—and found some striking differences. Compared with cartilage from disease-free people, cartilage from patients with osteoarthritis contained more water (making cartilage softer and more fragile), higher levels of cartilage-destroying enzymes, and scantier amounts of proteoglycans, the molecules so vital for cartilage resilience.

The dietary supplement glucosamine may work against osteoarthritis, and perhaps even help prevent it, by replenishing the proteoglycans inside cartilage.

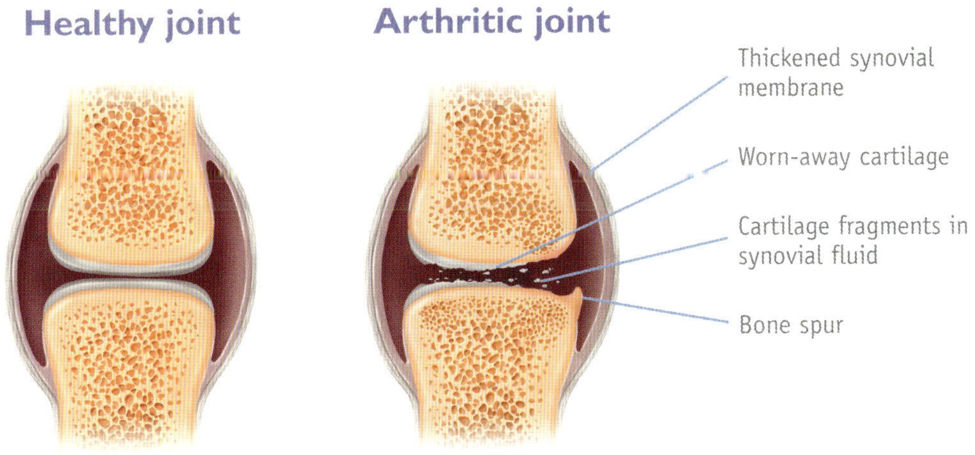

In a healthy joint (left), the bones are capped by smooth cartilage. The surrounding joint capsule has an inner lining that produces synovial fluid, which helps to lubricate the joint.

In a joint with osteoarthritis (right), the cartilage has become roughened and partially worn away. Chunks of broken-off cartilage have irritated the synovial membrane, making it inflamed and thickened. Loss of cartilage has increased pressure on the bones, which have formed spurs (osteophytes) around their edges.

BONING UP: If you have arthritis, there is a scientific name—crepitus—for the creaky feeling (and creaky noises) that you may notice when you move affected joints. Doctors feel for and listen for signs of crepitus when diagnosing arthritis in patients.

that maintain the structure of cartilage. With its collagen "superstructure" damaged, cartilage swells with water, becoming softer and more vulnerable to stresses that wear it away. Researchers have identified several risk factors that can significantly increase a person's odds of developing the disease:

Age

Age is clearly the most powerful predictor of whether a person develops osteoarthritis. The condition is rare in young people, but becomes increasingly more common in older age

on the horizon

As they seek the underlying cause of osteoarthritis, researchers are expanding their search beyond cartilage and into the underlying bone. Accumulating evidence suggests that changes in bone "turnover"—the counterbalancing process of bone synthesis and bone breakdown—may be involved in causing osteoarthritis. "Indeed, the cartilage may be the innocent bystander of a disease process that is centered more in bone than in cartilage," the British researcher Paul Dieppe has written.

what the studies show

A study of former U.S. football players found that more than 80 percent of players with a history of a knee injury had evidence of osteoarthritis 10 to 30 years after their careers had ended.

groups. But don't misunderstand: OA correlates with age, it isn't caused by it.

Instead, it now appears that factors associated with aging—and quite a few other factors as well—can make people susceptible to OA and cause their condition to worsen. Fortunately, we will show you how to reduce all these risk factors in later chapters.

Too many pounds

Wisdom isn't the only thing that increases with age. So does the waistline. Carrying around extra pounds puts constant stress on the joints that eventually damages the cartilage. This is particularly true for the weight-bearing joints: the knees and, to a lesser extent, the hips.

If you're overweight, losing those pounds is one of the most effective of all osteoarthritis treatments available. A study that followed women of different weights over 36 years found that the heaviest women (those in the upper 20 percent by weight) were more than three times likelier than women in the bottom 20 percent to develop severe osteoarthritis of the knee. This was the first study showing that OA may be prevented.

Loose joints

When the bones of a joint aren't bound tightly to each other, they can bang together and damage their protective cartilage. Such "joint instability" is now recognized as a major cause of the pain and early-morning stiffness that may occur long before cartilage damage has begun. (Such symptoms are often felt by young, "double-jointed" women whose flexibility makes them talented ballet dancers.) As a preventive measure, people with loose joints may be advised to avoid activities that could increase their risk of developing osteoarthritis prematurely.

On-the-job exertion

Certain jobs increase a person's risk for developing osteoarthritis. For example, OA of the knee is common among miners, dockworkers, and others who must constantly bend their knees or do heavy lifting on the job.

Look to your genes

In 1990, after studying a family whose members developed osteoarthritis in many of their joints at a very early age, researchers reported on the first "osteoarthritis gene." They traced OA to a gene responsible for making the collagen in cartilage. A mutation in this gene causes defective collagen to be produced, which probably weakens cartilage and causes it to break down prematurely.

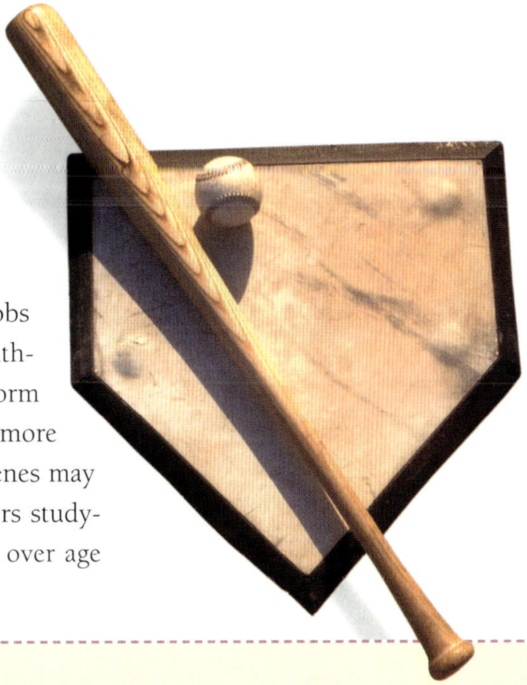

Genes seem to influence osteoarthritis in particular joints as well. In 1944, researchers reported that OA involving the end joints of the fingers was an inherited trait. In this condition, small bony knobs known as Heberden's nodes (named after the eighteenth-century British physician who first described them) form on the top of the finger joints. Heberden's nodes are more common in women, particularly after menopause. Genes may also influence OA in other joints. In 1998, researchers studying 616 pairs of identical and fraternal female twins over age

Arthritis Profile

Mickey Mantle

In the 1951 World Series, at the end of his rookie year, 20-year-old Mickey Mantle was playing right field for the New York Yankees. He was chasing a fly ball hit by the New York Giant's Willie Mays when his spikes caught on the cover of a drain pipe buried in the outfield turf. He tore the ligaments in his right knee, and his season was over.

Mantle's knee was operated on a few days later, but he never fully recovered from the injury. By trying to compensate for his painful right knee, he put more of his weight on his left knee and eventually damaged it as well.

Mantle's painful knees caused him to retire from baseball in 1969. The pain continued into retirement, and Mantle found he could no longer play golf or even climb the stairs.

Not until 1987 did Mantle learn the cause of his increasing infirmity: osteoarthritis. He was then prescribed nonsteroidal anti-inflammatory drugs, which had a dramatically beneficial effect on his condition. The pain and stiffness eased, stairs gave him much less trouble, and he could once again play 18 holes of golf.

Can You Run Away from Osteoarthritis?

If repetitive stresses can lead to osteoarthritis, are recreational runners at risk? Numerous studies have tried to answer this question, with decidedly mixed results.

Point and counterpoint. A 1996 study looked for signs of osteoarthritis in a group of former elite female athletes (67 middle- and long-distance runners and 14 tennis players) and in a control group of women of the same age from the general population. The ex-athletes were two to three times more likely than women in the control group to have osteoarthritis of the knees and hips. And a study published last year found that men under 50 who regularly run more than 20 miles per week faced an increased risk for osteoarthritis of the knee or hip.

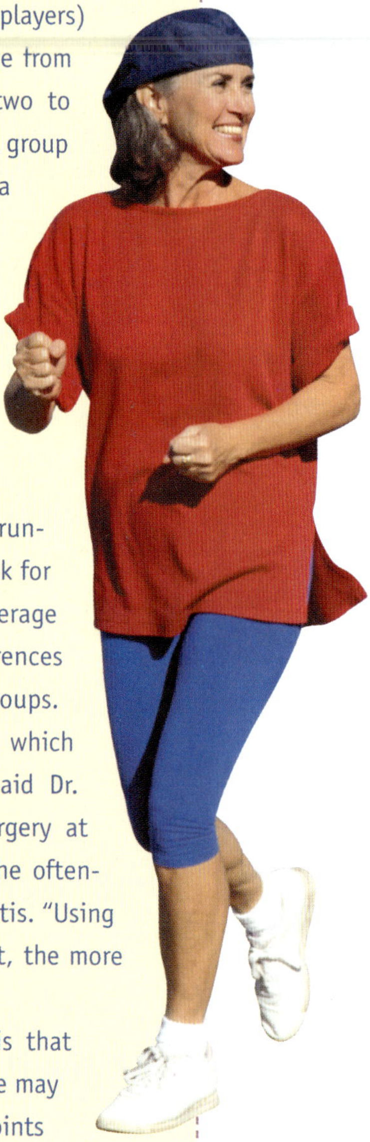

But other studies, involving amateur marathoners and other recreational runners, have found no link between running and osteoarthritis. One study, comparing 17 male runners who had run an average of 28 miles per week for 12 years with nonrunning men the same average weight and age (56 years old), found no differences in osteoarthritis prevalence between the two groups.

"Joints aren't like the bearings on your car, which wear out after a certain number of miles," said Dr. Joseph Buckwalter, professor of orthopedic surgery at the University of Iowa, in his 1998 review of the often-conflicting literature on athletics and osteoarthritis. "Using the joints doesn't necessarily hurt them—in fact, the more you use them, the better off you may be."

Bottom line. The consensus among experts is that recreational running or other high-impact exercise may accelerate osteoarthritis in previously damaged joints or when done strenuously for a number of years. Runners with healthy joints have less cause for worry, but probably shouldn't overdo it.

40 concluded that genetic factors may be responsible for half of all cases of OA of the hip.

Being a woman doesn't help

Women stand a much greater chance of developing osteoarthritis than men, especially as they get older. This gender difference is most extreme for OA of the knee in older people: Women over 65 are more than twice as likely to develop it as men the same age.

Couch potatoing

People tend to exercise less as they age—especially if they have arthritis. What's less well appreciated is that inactivity itself increases your risk for osteoarthritis in several ways:

- Inactivity leads to weight gain that puts extra strain on the joints.
- Tissues vital to joint movement—especially the muscles—can atrophy due to inactivity. Studies have shown that people with weak thigh muscles are more likely to develop OA of the knee.
- Inactivity can kill off chondrocytes, the cells that make and repair cartilage. Because cartilage has no blood vessels, chondrocytes must obtain nutrients from the synovial fluid. Walking or other weight-bearing activities contract and expand cartilage with each repetition, creating the pumping action of fluid vital for chondrocytes.

Taking a blow

The sports pages regularly report on athletes who've sustained serious injury to a joint—most often the knee. Unfortunately, an athlete or anyone else who suffers an injury to some part of

caution

Early diagnosis and treatment is the best approach for any type of osteoarthritis—but is especially important for osteoarthritis of the knee. Treatment—including drugs, weight loss, exercise, injections of hyaluronic acid, and walking aids—can all help prevent further joint damage. If left untreated, OA of the knee can become disabling, with joint replacement surgery the only recourse for a patient.

Do You Have Osteoarthritis? Surveil Your Symptoms

- One or more joints has a deep and aching pain that is steady or intermittent
- Pain is worsened by exercise or other activities and eased by rest
- Joint pain develops that won't go away, even after resting the joint for several days
- One or more joints feels stiff for 30 minutes or less after you get out of bed
- One or more joints swells or feels tender
- Affected joint has grinding feeling or makes a grinding sound
- When you start moving after sitting during the day—after driving a fairly long distance or seeing a movie, for example—you feel stiff for the next 20 or 30 minutes

a joint—cartilage, bone, ligament, or tendon—may eventually develop OA in that joint. With some injuries, such as a compound fracture of the ankle, osteoarthritis is almost a certainty. Many professional athletes who incur frequent knee injuries will develop OA of the knee after their playing days are over.

Joint by Joint: The Prime Targets of OA

Osteoarthritis can affect any of the body's joints, but it most often occurs in the hands, knees, hips, or spine.

Hands. Osteoarthritis of the fingers is usually hereditary. Heberden's nodes, the small bony knobs that form on the ends of finger joints, occur most often in middle-aged and older women. The nodes are usually painless and tend to develop so slowly over many years that a woman may not notice them until, for example, she has trouble slipping a ring over the joint.

Heberden's nodes are twice as likely to develop in women

whose mothers also have them. Similar enlargements on the middle finger joints are known as Bouchard's nodes. Both Heberden's and Bouchard's nodes may first develop in one or a few fingers and later affect others. As Heberden himself noted, the problem with these nodes is mainly cosmetic.

A more painful form of OA affecting the end joints of fingers is called nodal osteoarthritis. A single joint suddenly becomes painful, tender, and swollen for three or four weeks—and then the problem subsides. Nodal OA is also hereditary and mainly affects women 45 and older, who are 10 times more likely to develop it than men in the same age group.

The joint at the base of the thumb also commonly develops osteoarthritis. By contrast, OA rarely affects the knuckles (where the fingers attach to the wrist).

caution

Joint pain that does not abate after a few days of rest is a clear signal that you should see a doctor soon.

Knees. The knees bear more weight than any other joint in the body—which makes them very susceptible to OA. When that happens, the knees may become swollen and feel stiff and painful when you try to move them. You may notice you have trouble walking to the mailbox, climbing stairs, and getting in and out of the car. According to studies, strengthening the muscles surrounding the knee can often dramatically improve the symptoms of osteoarthritis of the knee.

Hips. Like the knees, the hips are weight-bearing joints and are likewise susceptible to OA. People with osteoarthritis of the hip may have trouble bending, and the pain and stiffness may cause them to limp when they walk. The pain may not only be felt in the hip but may also "radiate" to other parts of the body, especially the groin or down the inside of the thigh. As we've already said, some cases of osteoarthritis of the hip seem to be hereditary. Also, people who are bowlegged or who have other congenital abnormalities that cause the bones of the hip to be misaligned are at increased risk for hip osteoarthritis.

Losing weight can help—but is not as helpful for relieving hip osteoarthritis as it is for the knee. Drugs and exercise can also help relieve pain and improve movement. Hip-replacement surgery is very effective when other treatments fall short of relieving the pain or disability.

Spine. Osteoarthritis of the spine mainly causes stiffness and pain in the neck or in the lower back. Measures that can help relieve the symptoms include exercises that strengthen the muscles of the back and abdomen; heat treatments; and use of support pillows when sitting. In some people, bone spurs growing from the edges of the vertebrae may squeeze the spinal nerves, causing pain, weakness, or numbness in the arms or legs. When this happens, surgery may be necessary to relieve the pressure on the nerves.

How Does OA Progress?

The breakdown of cartilage that leads to OA doesn't occur overnight—although that first sharp pain in your hip or knee may make you think it does. This erosion almost always occurs slowly, over many months or years, as the once-smooth and slippery cartilage becomes thinner, develops a roughened surface, and loses its cushioning ability.

Similarly, the pain and stiffness that accompany the disintegrating cartilage may appear so gradually that many people ignore it or chalk it up to "getting older." And for many lucky people, this is as far as osteoarthritis ever progresses: It remains a mild problem, causing symptoms they're barely aware of.

> "Joints aren't like the bearings on your car, which wear out after a certain number of miles. The more you use them, the better off you may be."
>
> — Dr. Joseph Buckwalter, University of Iowa

When cartilage continues eroding, however, people may begin experiencing the bothersome symptoms that eventually send them to the doctor's office. After exercise, knees and other joints may ache or feel stiff for a brief time. You may also feel stiff after you've been sitting for awhile—when climbing out of the car after a long ride, for example, or getting up after watching a movie.

Bone meets bone. Eventually, cartilage wears away to the point that, in some areas, bone rubs against bone. People may feel their knees briefly "lock" as they climb stairs or may experience a grinding sensation—or even hear a grinding sound—when they bend affected knees or hips. People may also find themselves avoiding once-routine activities that now cause pain—the daily walk to the newsstand, for example, or working in the garden on weekends. If the affected joint is a hip or knee, people may begin to limp as they try to minimize the pain.

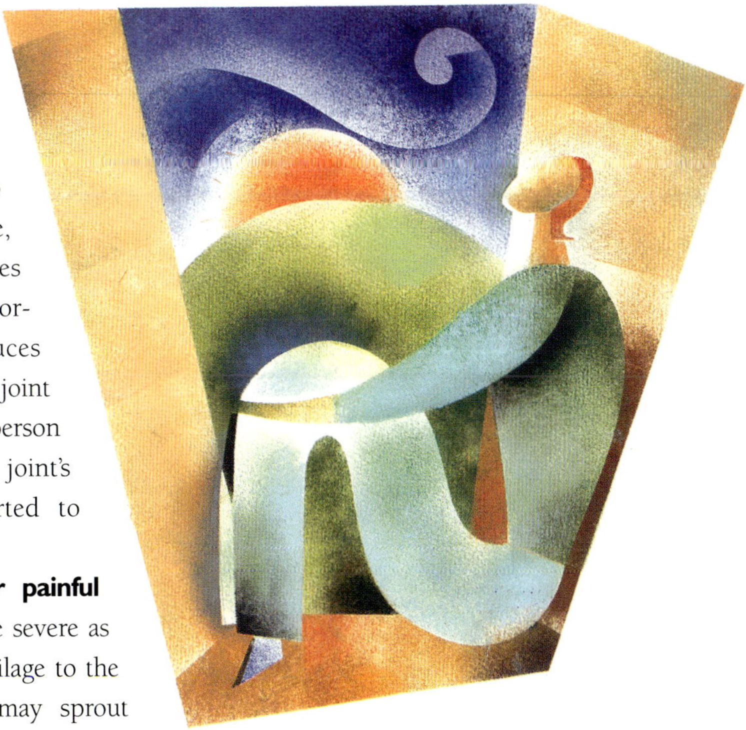

Small chunks of fragmented cartilage floating in the synovial fluid may be irritating the synovial membrane and adding to the discomfort; in response, the membrane becomes inflamed, painful, and abnormally thick, and produces excess fluid that makes the joint swell. In addition to pain, a person may now notice that the joint's range of motion has started to become restricted.

Bone spurs and other painful growths. OA becomes more severe as changes extend beyond cartilage to the underlying bones, which may sprout small growths (known as bone spurs or osteophytes) around their outer edges. Bone spurs increase the joint's surface area and may be the bones' defensive reaction to the extra pressure created when their protective covering has worn away.

Unfortunately, bone spurs often make things worse: Spurs on the spine, for example, may cause severe pain by pinching nerves connecting the spinal cord to the muscles, and sharp spurs that form around the rim of the knee joint may worsen the pain and tenderness. By this time, people may find that arthritis pain is keeping them awake at night.

When cartilage is completely eroded, the sensitive bones rub against each other within the joint. At this point, the pain from osteoarthritis can be excruciating and nearly unrelenting even after the slightest movement. When such severe osteoarthritis affects the weight-bearing joints—the knees or the hips—it can be crippling, especially if:

- Uneven cartilage loss has created uneven joint surfaces, causing bones to become misaligned and leading to instability in the joint itself.

- Extensive bone-spur formation limits a joint's mobility.

did you know

Osteoarthritis pain tends to worsen toward the end of the day. In many other types of arthritis, pain remains constant during the day or is worse in the morning.

- Because of disuse, muscles and tendons that support the joint have shortened and weakened, leading to muscle spasms and even more disability. As noted later, today's joint-replacement operations can be a godsend for people with such severe osteoarthritis.

How Is OA Diagnosed?

Relief for your pain means getting your health problem diagnosed accurately so that treatment can begin. For doctors familiar with OA, telling whether you have the disease usually isn't difficult. The diagnosis is based on taking your clinical history, doing a physical exam, and running some tests.

Clinical history

The doctor will ask you a series of questions to get information about your symptoms—when they started, where they occur,

Getting Your Doc Up to Speed

Taking your medical history at the initial visit is a crucial part of the diagnostic process, since it can help your doctor determine what type of arthritis you have and choose the right laboratory tests to confirm the diagnosis. You can do your doctor and yourself a big favor by arriving well prepared. Try to bring:

- Your medical records, including copies of recent X rays and blood tests
- A list of other medical problems that you have
- A list of all the drugs you take—prescription and over-the-counter as well as herbs or other dietary supplements
- A written "narrative" in which you describe your problem as fully as you can, including: how long ago the joint pain began, whether the symptoms came on suddenly or slowly, which joints were initially affected, what triggered the symptoms (e.g., exercise, climbing stairs, etc.), and the activities that your joint pain interferes with.

what they feel like, whether they've changed over time, how they're affecting your life. The doctor will also ask about other diseases you may have (which could be the cause of your symptoms) and drugs you may be taking (which may interfere with anti-arthritis drugs that may be recommended).

caution

If your doctor skimps on either the conversation or the physical examination and attempts to diagnose or rule out osteoarthritis on the basis of X rays alone, find yourself another doctor.

Doctors have found that answers to three questions in particular provide a good gauge of whether a patient has arthritis or some other musculoskeletal disease and how severely disabled he or she is:

- Do you have any pain or stiffness in your muscles, joints, or back?
- Can you dress yourself completely without any difficulty?
- Can you walk up and down stairs without any difficulty?

The doctor then follows up any positive answers with more specific questions. The discussion should also cover:

- **Pain:** The location of the pain, its severity, character, timing.
- **Stiffness:** No other condition causes the same type of joint stiffness as osteoarthritis.
- **Swelling:** Eighty-five to 90 percent of people with osteoarthritis don't experience swelling. However, swelling can indicate the degree of joint damage or suggest that there's another problem.
- **Severity:** The degree of pain suggests joint damage and how much treatment you may need.
- **Causes:** Knowing if you suffered an injury before the pain started is a valuable clue that you are suffering from secondary OA. If no injury occurred, chances increase that you have primary osteoarthritis.

The physical exam

Following a routine exam to assess your overall health (taking your blood pressure, listening to your heart), the doctor will focus on the joints that are bothering you—feeling and pressing on them for signs of swelling or tenderness and watching how they "work" when you walk or bend. The doctor will also assess other joints, which could be affected by arthritis even though you don't know it yet.

During the joint examination, the doctor will ask you to move joints ("active motion") and will also move them himself ("passive motion"). In true joint disease, movement is limited and causes pain with both active and passive motion. If the doctor can move a joint further than you can (flex your knee in a wider arc, for example), then you probably don't have a problem with your joint but instead with the tendons or muscles surrounding it.

Different joints are examined in different ways:

Hands. The doctor checks for bony enlargements on the end joints of fingers or on the middle joints. These outgrowths, or nodes, are clear signs of osteoarthritis.

Hips. Limited range of motion is the key indicator. With the patient lying on his back with knees bent, the doctor places one hand on the knee and the other on the heel and then rotates the foot outward and inward. Restricted inward rotation is typically an early sign of hip osteoarthritis.

Knees. In addition to checking for abnormalities in joint movement, the doctor looks for areas of swelling around the knee joint.

Spine. The doctor palpates (feels) the contours of the spine to check for abnormal tenderness and assesses range of motion—whether the patient can touch his ear with his shoulder, for example.

Lab tests

Blood tests. Osteoarthritis can almost always be diagnosed without the need for laboratory tests, which are routinely normal in osteoarthritis patients. The main reason for laboratory tests is to rule out other possible diseases such as rheumatoid arthritis. For this reason, some doctors routinely order two blood tests for all patients with painful joints: the rheumatoid factor test and erythrocyte sedimentation. These tests, discussed in more detail on pages 66-67, can help to indicate whether rheumatoid arthritis is present.

Analyzing joint fluid. Taking a sample of synovial fluid,

did you know

Bones and bone spurs can be seen on X rays, but cartilage can't because it doesn't contain calcium salts. So cartilage essentially is visualized by its absence: In a normal joint, the black and apparently blank space separating two bones is the cartilage at the ends of the bones. As osteoarthritis progresses, X rays show this "blank" space increasingly narrowing as more cartilage is lost and the bones get closer together and, perhaps, eventually touch.

removed from the joint with a needle, also helps rule out other possible health problems. Abnormally high levels of white blood cells indicate inflammation and the presence of several possible conditions—including gout, inflammatory types of arthritis such as rheumatoid arthritis or psoriatic arthritis, or arthritis due to an infection (septic arthritis). As a bonus, draining fluid from a joint can help relieve pressure and pain in a joint.

X rays

These aren't really useful in diagnosing osteoarthritis, since a significant amount of cartilage must be lost before the damage shows up on an X ray. But X rays in someone known to have osteoarthritis can reveal the extent of the damage. They can show how much cartilage has been lost, whether underlying bone has been damaged, or whether bone spurs are present. In addition, X rays taken periodically can monitor the progression of osteoarthritis.

Strange but true. Interestingly, the severity of a person's symptoms may be totally unrelated to how the joint looks on an X ray. In fact, only one third of people whose X rays show the presence of osteoarthritis report pain or any other symptoms. On the other hand, some people whose joints look perfectly normal on an X ray may have excruciating symptoms from osteoarthritis.

Another imaging technique—magnetic resonance imaging, or MRI—excels at revealing injuries to soft tissues such as muscles and tendons. But so far, MRI has no advantage over X rays in evaluating or monitoring joints affected by osteoarthritis.

What Now?

Learning that you have a chronic disease can be disturbing, and a diagnosis of osteoarthritis is no exception. Are you destined for a life of constant pain? Can you continue working, traveling, playing with your grandchildren, or otherwise living life like before? The answers are largely reassuring: OA is not a disease that you need to dread.

The good news. Even when severe, osteoarthritis is limited to the joints and won't affect your heart, brain, or other parts of the body. And today, the great majority of people with OA can be effectively treated—their pain and stiffness eased and their joint

on the horizon

A new procedure developed in Sweden involves removing a sample of healthy cartilage and sending it to a laboratory for cultivation. When millions of cells have grown, surgeons remove the damaged cartilage and replace it with lab-grown cartilage. Newer still is an operation in which a small amount of cartilage and bone is removed from the leg, ground up, and placed in the damaged joint, where it stimulates cartilage growth.

movement improved—with a combination of anti-inflammatory drugs, exercise, rest, moist heat, and the take-charge approach to arthritis described in this book.

Surgical solutions. When pain and immobility from hip or knee osteoarthritis can't be relieved in any other way, surgical joint replacement may be necessary. Fortunately, over the past 20 years, medical science has made great advances in joint-replacement surgery, and most people with severe arthritis can look forward to dramatic improvements after undergoing it—free of pain and able to function nearly as well as before their osteoarthritis developed.

did you know

The aerobic exercises that pose the least risk of damaging joints are swimming, cycling, and walking.

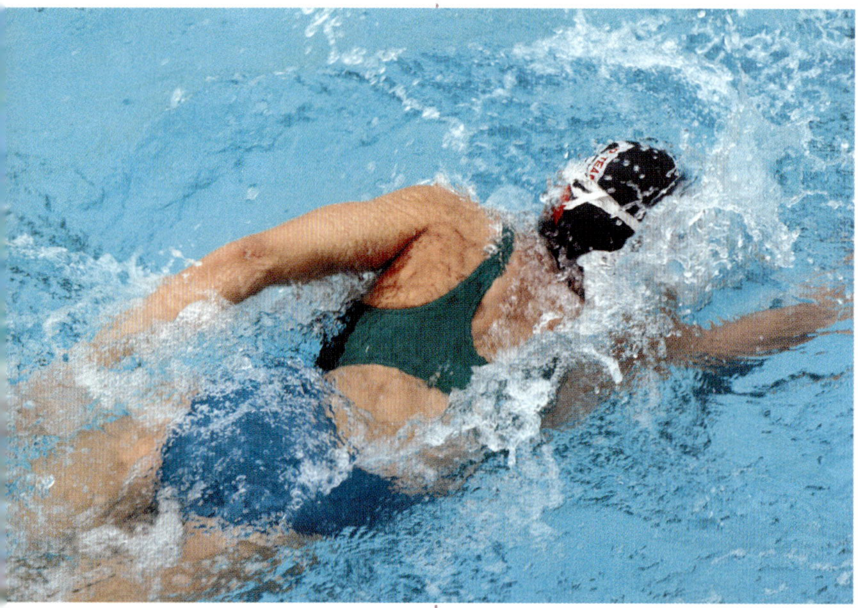

How Is OA Treated?

There's no need to let arthritis take charge of your life. Instead, you have the power to take charge of it. Virtually all cases of osteoarthritis respond to treatments to ease your pain and stiffness, keep you active and productive, protect and strengthen affected joints, and prevent symptoms from worsening.

To achieve those results, you need to work with your doctor to develop an individual action plan. This plan will take into account the severity of your symptoms, the joints that are affected, your age, the limitations on your daily activities, and other health problems you may have. For many people, a combination of several of the following therapies works best. All will be discussed more fully in later chapters.

Lose it

Being overweight puts extra stress on your weight-bearing joints—especially the knees and hips. If you're overweight and have osteoarthritis, losing those pounds could dramatically improve your symptoms.

Heat it up, cool it down

Heat applied with a hot-water bottle, hot towels, hot packs, a hot shower, or a heating pad can be a very effective treatment for the pain and stiffness of OA. For unknown reasons, moist heat seems to provide the greatest relief. Heat can also be administered as deep or penetrating heat in office procedures that use diathermy or ultrasound devices. Cold is most useful for joints that are acutely inflamed—which is rarely a problem in osteoarthritis.

Move it

Doctors once advised their osteoarthritis patients against exercising, believing that exercise could further damage their joints. But research over the past decade has found that exercise ranks as one of the best treatments for osteoarthritis. The proper exercises can relieve pain, improve flexibility, and help you in your weight-loss efforts. As a bonus, exercising will enhance your overall health by reducing stress, lowering your risk for heart disease, diabetes, and several types of cancer.

Swallow it

A wide variety of drugs, both over-the-counter and prescription, can help ease the vexing symptoms of OA. They include the pain reliever acetaminophen (Tylenol), topical or rub-on pain relievers (especially useful for the knee and fingers), and nonsteroidal anti-inflammatory drugs such as ibuprofen (Advil, Nuprin) and naproxen (Aleve). The NSAIDs relieve pain as well as inflammation that may be present. Three recently approved NSAIDs—Celebrex, Vioxx, and Mobic—are much less likely to cause bleeding and other gastrointestinal side effects.

Hyaluronic acid injections

People with osteoarthritis of the knee who haven't been helped by NSAIDs or other pain relievers have a new treatment option: injections of hyaluronic acid, a natural substance found in synovial fluid that helps lubricate the joint. The procedure is called visco-supplementation. The jelly-like hyaluronic acid is injected weekly into the knee for three to five weeks. In clinical studies, these injections have proved as effec-

what the studies show

In one animal study, something called cartilage growth factor was combined with fibrinogen, which acts as a glue to hold the growth factor to damaged cartilage. Various concentrations of this mixture were inserted into the joints of several groups of animals. A year later the animals had formed new cartilage.

caution

All NSAIDs are basically equal in effectiveness, but in practice, OA patients can respond poorly to one and very well to another. You may have to try several before finding the one that works best for you.

tive as continual NSAID therapy in providing pain relief that can last for months.

Injected steroids

Injecting steroids directly into a painful joint can temporarily relieve pain and inflammation. Steroids are generally prescribed for an intense flare-up of pain and inflammation or if a patient doesn't find relief from other painkillers. This short-term measure should not be done more than two or three times per year because of the risk of side effects.

Rheumatism: Gone But Not Forgotten

The word *rheumatism* isn't used much anymore, but its origins can be traced all the way back to the ancient Greek theory of disease.

Until about 100 years ago, what we now know as arthritis was mainly referred to as *rheumatism*, a word probably coined in the second century A.D. by Galen, the illustrious Greek physician. The Greeks believed that diseases were caused by four primary substances, or humors, that flowed from the brain to various parts of the body. Diseases occurred at the places in the body where these flows stopped. The Greek word *rheuma* means flux and referred to the slow-flowing humor that afflicted the joints and caused pain, swelling, and stiffness. Through the following centuries, *rheumatism* became a broadly used term for aches and pains anywhere in the body.

Today, doctors rarely call a patient's problem *rheumatism*, but instead diagnose it as a particular type of arthritis. Nevertheless, *rheuma* remains firmly entrenched in arthritis lingo. Rheumatology was created in 1949 as the medical specialty for the study of joint diseases, and its practitioners are rheumatologists; *The Journal of Rheumatology* is a leading publication for highlighting studies on joint diseases; rheumatoid arthritis is a well-known type of arthritis; and an important class of drugs for treating RA is the disease-modifying anti-rheumatic drugs, or DMARDs.

Surgery

Surgeons can make small repairs to cartilage with an arthroscope—a long viewing tube inserted through small incisions in the skin. Arthroscopy can help alleviate the symptoms of osteoarthritis, but unfortunately it cannot stop the progression of the disease.

Surgery can also help osteoarthritis by preventing the joint from becoming deformed or even correcting an existing deformity; removing part of the bone around the joint to allow for movement; replacing a damaged joint with an artificial joint made of plastic, metal, or ceramic; immobilizing a joint to correct severe joint problems.

Alternative treatments

Several dietary supplements (glucosamine, chondroitin sulfate and SAM-e) show promise in osteoarthritis—not only for relieving pain but also for rebuilding cartilage. In addition, studies show that adequate intake of several vitamins including C, E and beta carotene may reduce your risk of developing osteoarthritis or—if you already have it—prevent it from worsening.

Rheumatoid Arthritis: Fire in the Joints

Rheumatoid arthritis (RA) is the most common type of inflammatory arthritis and usually affects many joints in the body. RA is much less common than osteoarthritis, affecting only about one percent of the U.S. population, or some 2.1 million people. Some 100,000 new cases of RA are diagnosed every year, with women accounting for three of every four people with the disease. RA can begin at any age, but most commonly develops in young and middle-age adults.

did you know

- Experts now believe that morning stiffness (also known as "gelling") results from the accumulation of synovial fluid inside the joint while the person with arthritis is asleep. Once the person wakes up and starts moving, the excess fluid is pumped out and the stiffness subsides.
- Scientists in several laboratories are experimenting with different formulations of synthetic cartilage or cartilage substitutes that might replace arthritis-damaged knee cartilage. Among the wide range of materials being studied are ground diamonds, ceramics, liquid polyurethane, and a new organic material called Salubria.

RA versus OA: Comparisons & Contrasts

Age of occurrence. Rheumatoid arthritis (RA) usually develops between the ages of 20 and 50, but can occur at any age. Osteoarthritis (OA) is a disease of middle and old age and rarely occurs before age 45.

Pattern of disease. RA often strikes symmetrically, meaning it affects both wrists, the knuckles on both hands, etc. OA rarely affects both joints (e.g., both wrists) at once.

Speed of onset. About 20 percent of RA cases develop suddenly, within weeks or months. OA develops slowly, with cartilage breakdown usually occurring over several years.

Extent of illness. In addition to causing joint damage, RA can cause fatigue, fever, anemia, and weight loss, and damage the heart and other organs. OA is limited to the joints.

Joints affected. RA usually affects many joints, including the wrists (affected in almost all RA patients), knuckles, elbows, shoulders, ankles, feet, and neck (but usually spares the rest of the spine). OA most commonly affects the knees, hips, feet, hands, and spine; sometimes affects the knuckles and wrists; and rarely affects the elbows and shoulders.

Hand involvement. RA affects many of the hand joints, but usually not the knuckles closest to the fingernails. OA affects the knuckles closest to the fingernails more often than other joints of the hand.

Morning stiffness. People with RA have prolonged morning stiffness, usually lasting for at least 30 minutes after they get up. With OA, morning stiffness lasts less than 30 minutes.

What Is RA?

RA is a systemic disease, meaning it can affect not only the joints but also the blood vessels, heart, skin, muscles, and other parts of the body. Most people with RA must contend with daily pain and stiffness that may wax and wane. They often speak of having good and bad days, weeks, or months, and of enduring periods of depression, anxiety, and helplessness. This book's self-empowerment approach has proved its usefulness in helping people with RA gain control over their disease and over their lives.

Boning Up: If you have arthritis, you may swear that your stiffness and pain get worse when the weather changes. They probably do. Studies using climate chambers have found that people with arthritis really do experience increased stiffness and pain when the barometric pressure drops quickly or when the humidity suddenly rises.

Do you really have it? RA and osteoarthritis are often mistaken for each other—which can cause serious problems, since the two types of arthritis are treated quite differently. Although symptoms may be similar, RA and OA are very different diseases.

Osteoarthritis can affect any joint that has cartilage—freely movable joints such as the knee or slightly movable joints like the vertebrae. By contrast, RA focuses on the body's freely movable joints and on one area in particular: the synovial membrane, which is the inner lining of the capsule surrounding freely movable joints. Once this joint becomes inflamed, the characteristic symptoms of rheumatoid arthritis—heat, swelling, stiffness, and pain—can then be felt.

While osteoarthritis confines its damage to the joints, RA is a systemic disease that can damage not only the joints but also other parts of the body such as blood vessels, the eyes, and the heart. This tissue damage is caused by chronic inflammation—the hallmark of RA. Although inflammation can also occur in osteoarthritis, it is confined to the affected joints.

What Causes RA?

The causes of RA's key feature—chronic inflammation—are not known. However, scientists do know that a glitch in the immune system is involved. Like psoriasis, lupus, multiple sclerosis, and

continued on page 62

on the horizon

A treatment that may actually cure rheumatoid arthritis was reported late last year at the annual scientific meeting of the American College of Rheumatology. Developed by researchers at University College in London, the new treatment involves depleting the blood of B lymphocytes; these immune cells form antibodies that cause much of the joint destruction that occurs in RA. The Arthritis Foundation described B lymphocyte depletion as "a promising new way of treating" RA and said these early results "show a magnitude of response in patients that far exceeds any other therapies we currently use to treat RA."

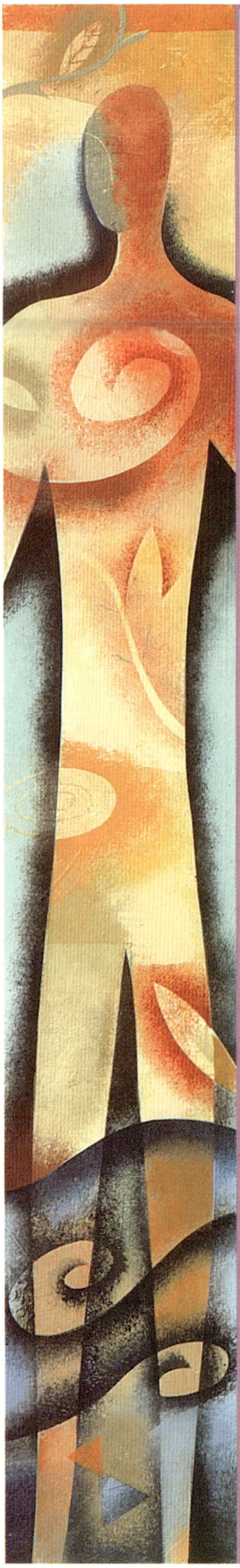

REAL-LIFE MEDICINE

Living with Rheumatoid Arthritis

Sharon Dorough clearly remembers her last carefree day. It was July 4, 1977, and she was working at a church camp in Alabama. Since staff members had off the Fourth of July, Sharon and several of her co-workers went to a nearby state park for a picnic. There they had a tree-climbing contest, which Sharon won—not surprising, since 18-year-old Sharon was a good athlete who had run distance events for her high school track team.

"The next morning, when I woke up, it had pretty much hit me from my neck down—my neck, my shoulders, elbows, wrists, hands, knees, hips, feet," Sharon recalls. "You could see the swelling—my knees were huge—and the joints were painful and stiff. It happened very dramatically and literally overnight."

Despite her condition, Sharon stuck with her summer job. "I was having fun, and I was away from home living with a bunch of other teenagers," she says. But she was also in constant pain: "I remember very vividly walking down the stairs from my room to the lobby in the building I stayed in and crying because each step hurt so much," she recalls.

Finally, about six weeks later, Sharon returned home to Gadsden, Alabama, for her sister's wedding. Her mother insisted she see a doctor, and Sharon was hospitalized for the medical tests that showed she had rheumatoid arthritis (RA).

Today, someone in Sharon's condition would immediately be placed on one or more of the potent disease-modifying antirheumatic drugs, or DMARDs, which slow down the process of RA. But Sharon's family doctor prescribed high-dose aspirin for her. A couple of years later, a rheumatologist did put her on injectable gold (see p. 154), one of the first DMARDs.

Sharon completed college at the University of Alabama at Tuscaloosa and took a job at an advertising agency in Birmingham, Alabama, where she now lives. But ultimately, her worsening arthritis forced her to stop working. "I was becoming more disabled every day," she recalls. "My left hip was degenerating pretty quickly, and even though I used a cane, I had to stay home most of the time because I wasn't able to get out and walk. And I couldn't sit at a desk and work at a computer because my neck was so stiff.

"It really was a tough period in my life, and I was very depressed, in part because I was told I needed hip replacement surgery," says Sharon. She qualified for Social Security disability and got handicapped parking tags for her car: "Driving to the grocery store and coming home was a big day for me," she says.

Before long, Sharon realized she needed to do something. "I got tired of sitting home feeling sorry for myself—that got old pretty fast," she says. She heard that the Arthritis Foundation's Self-Help Course was being offered at her church, signed up for it in 1990—and began turning her life around.

You could see the swelling—my knees were huge—and the joints were painful and stiff.

Sharon ultimately taught the course herself, and last year she was certified as a course leader who trains other teachers. She serves on the local and chapter board of the Arthritis Foundation and on the national board of the foundation's American Juvenile Arthritis Organization.

"The self-help course was a turning point for me because it changed the way I thought about having arthritis," says Sharon. "I stopped viewing myself as a victim. Instead, while I might not be able to handle the way my body reacts to the disease, I realized that I can handle the way I react to my body. And this shift in attitude has made a really big difference in my life."

One way the self-help course changes attitudes, says Sharon, is by emphasizing "contracting," where participants set goals and then try to fulfill them. "When I took the course I hated doing the contracting, but now I realize its importance," says Sharon. "It enables people to discover that they have it within themselves to take charge of their disease. This is power they didn't know they had, and it allows them to do things they didn't know were possible."

A contract, says Sharon, has "a very specific, measurable goal." You say what you are going to do, when you are going to do it, and the distance or length of time involved. "For example," she says, "I contracted to walk one mile

continued on page 60

REAL-LIFE MEDICINE *CONTINUED*

three times a week after supper. Or if your goal is to limit caffeine intake, you might contract to limit your coffee consumption to two cups a day. Then you come back the next week and report on whether you fulfilled your contract. You also have that extra incentive of peer-group pressure, since you don't want to have to say, 'Well, I was real lazy this week, I didn't do anything.'"

The course, says Sharon, also changed her approach to doctor visits. "It seems kind of comical now, but I remember early on that I'd go to the doctor to see how I was doing—as if I didn't know my body well enough to judge whether I was feeling bad or good. After taking the self-help course, I realized it was far better to tell the doctor how I was doing rather than the other way around. But that's a real change of perspective for most people—especially women, since we were brought up to be more accepting of authority."

In describing her own passivity before she took the self-help course, Sharon says: "To be honest, I'm not even sure what drugs I was on—I didn't keep track. I just took the pills that my doctor told me to take and when he told me to take them.

"One of the big things I got out of the course was that it was okay to ask questions," says Sharon. "In fact, you should be asking questions—and if you don't, you're probably dumber than you think you are! I've learned to write down my questions before I go in for a doctor visit, because I know that I'm not going to think them up once I'm there."

"If a drug isn't working... don't wait six months, but instead tell the doctor immediately."

Asking the *right* questions and getting satisfactory answers is also crucial, Sharon says. "At best nowadays, you'll probably have about 10 minutes with your doctor, so you have to make the most of your time. One of the things I hear so much from self-help course participants is 'we didn't have nearly enough time left to ask my important questions, and I still don't know what I'm supposed to do.'

"To prevent those problems,

we try to get people to role-play, so they'll get used to being more assertive about asking questions—asking the important ones first and making sure they get satisfactory answers. And if a drug isn't working or is causing stomach upset, for example, don't wait until you come back in six months, but instead tell the doctor immediately," Sharon says.

"I suspect that some people who hear about the self-help course decide not to take it because they don't want to get into that 'poor pitiful me' role," Sharon adds. "But the course is really not like that at all. We do talk about things that make us angry and frustrated, but we also discuss how to deal with those problems and get past them. I think the people who take the course and learn its techniques become much stronger people because of it."

In 1991, Sharon had the hip-replacement surgery that she had been dreading—and found that it "made a huge difference in my life. I was able to get around so much better." Unfortunately, her new right hip developed a problem and had to be replaced again five years later.

"Now," she says, "my other hip is going out—it's getting pretty close to having no cartilage—but I'm still functional. By now I'm very good at modifying my activities to fit how I feel that day. I can't do what most people would think of as normal activities, but I can do what, for me, is normal."

Sharon has learned that coping successfully with arthritis means having a positive attitude and being willing to make adjustments. "The way I figure it, you either learn to manage your arthritis or you lose the battle," she says. "It's much better to be positive about what you can do in spite of your arthritis than to dwell on what you can't do anymore.

"For example, I would love to go hiking and backpacking and engage in other strenuous activities," says Sharon. "But I know that if I do, my chances of doing something that will mess up my knees, hips, or other joints are high. Since I'm in this for the long haul, I avoid those activities and instead get my exercise through walking and swimming."

Sharon sums up her approach this way: "Living smarter with arthritis means conserving your energy for what's most important in your life, and then pacing yourself."

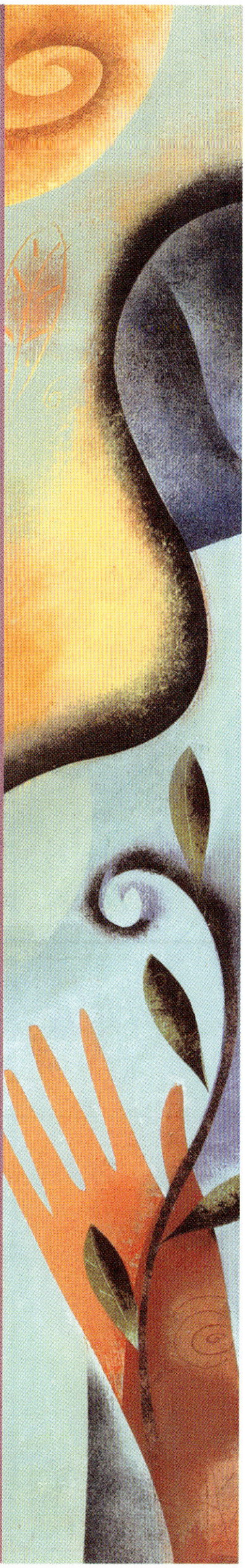

type I diabetes, RA is an autoimmune disease, meaning that the body's immune system mistakenly attacks healthy tissue as if it were a foreign invader.

Boning Up: Rheumatoid arthritis can affect any of the body's freely movable joints, but most commonly involves the hands, wrists, shoulders, elbows, knees, ankles, and feet.

RA's target. This autoimmune attack is directed against the joint's synovial membrane. It inflames the joint and causes pain, warmth, stiffness, and swelling—symptoms common to many types of arthritis. What distinguishes RA from all other forms of inflammatory arthritis is the potential for the inflamed synovial membrane to severely damage the joints.

In addition, RA's inflammation may spread beyond the joints to affect other parts of the body. Fortunately, new disease-modifying drugs can block this destructive inflammation by inactivating the immune system components that attack the body's own tissues.

Researchers have identified risk factors that make some people more likely to develop RA than others. Chief among these risk factors is a person's genetic makeup.

did you know

Nearly 90 percent of the joints that are ultimately affected in RA will be affected during the first year of the disease. So if you've had RA for several years, there is the consolation of knowing that the disease probably won't spread any further.

The role of heredity

People who develop RA do seem to inherit a susceptibility to the disease. Several different genes probably determine whether someone will have a tendency to develop RA and how severe his or her disease will be. As you might expect, these tend to be genes that control immune system function.

For example, some 65 percent of people with RA have a genetic marker—a protein called HLA-DR4—on the surface of their white blood cells. White cells play major roles in the body's effort to fight infections, so this protein may somehow "mislead" white cells into attacking the body's own tissues.

A missing link. Patients who have this genetic marker usually have more severe RA than those patients without it. However, fully one in four people who have the marker never develop RA, which shows that having "RA genes" isn't sufficient to bring on the condition. Instead, researchers believe something must be present to trigger RA in susceptible people.

The search for a trigger. For nearly a century, researchers have searched for a link between dozens of infectious agents and the development of RA. Bacteria have long been prime suspects: Since they were implicated in causing some types of arthritis, such as Reiter's syndrome, it made sense that bacteria could be involved in RA as well.

In 1912, an American rheumatologist proposed that RA occurred when bacterial toxins from localized infections in the tonsils, gums, teeth, or gallbladder were carried to the joins via the bloodstream. This "focal infection" theory failed to hold water, but for the next 30 years unfortunate RA patients had their tonsils removed or all their teeth pulled in a vain effort to halt the progress of the disease.

To see if RA was contagious, researchers in 1950 took fluid from the joints of people with RA and injected it into the joints of healthy volunteers. None of the volunteers developed RA—conclusive evidence that RA does not involve a persistent infection of the joints.

In recent years, viruses have received the most attention as possible culprits in triggering RA. A prime suspect for more than a decade has been the Epstein-Barr virus, which causes mononucleosis. Studies show that susceptible people—those with any one of three genes associated with RA—tend to have an abnormal immune response to Epstein-Barr infections that may trigger RA.

Many arthritis experts remain convinced that infections can initiate RA. So far, the strenuous efforts to link a bacterium, virus, or some other infectious agent to the condition have all failed. But even if some microbe eventually is implicated in causing RA, one thing seems certain: You can't "catch" RA from someone else.

The estrogen factor

Women are much more susceptible to autoimmune diseases than men—and RA is no exception: Three of every four people who develop RA are women, and researchers suspect the hormone estrogen. Combined with certain "susceptibility genes," estrogen seems to tip the balance toward developing RA: For example, a

what the studies show

A study published in 2000 supports the notion that Epstein-Barr infections could play a role in some cases of RA. Comparing 55 people with RA to people without, researchers from the University of Gottingen in Germany found that RA patients had double the levels of antibody against Epstein-Barr as people without RA. In addition, 14 of the RA patients had evidence of a reactivated Epstein-Barr infection compared with none of those without RA.

woman who inherits the genes will very likely develop the disease, while a brother with the same genes will remain healthy. When a woman has a genetic tendency to develop RA, estrogen may super-sensitize her immune system so that—in response to some infection—immune cells launch an attack on her tissues and the invading microbes.

How Does RA Progress?

In about 80 percent of cases, RA begins slowly, affecting just a few joints at first, typically those in the fingers, wrists, or toes. Eventually, the disease almost always ends up affecting 20 joints or more, including the shoulders, ankles, hips, knees, and other joints. But not all cases develop gradually: RA sometimes appears seemingly overnight, involving many of the body's joints in just a matter of days.

If this inflammation of a joint's synovial membrane persists, the membrane's cells may begin growing uncontrollably, forming extra tissue called pannus and thickening the normally thin membrane. The joint becomes swollen and feels puffy to the touch.

A slow cascade of pain. As RA progresses, the growing synovial membrane spreads and eventually covers the top of the joint cartilage. Invading cells from the thickened, inflamed synovial membrane release destructive enzymes that erode the cartilage and underlying bone of the joint and eventually weaken the muscles, tendons, and ligaments that surround it.

In the later stages of RA, joints become so severely damaged that they can no longer function properly. The inflammation may totally erode the cartilage and deform a joint by causing bones to fuse together. Fortunately, today's disease-modifying anti-rheumatic drugs can prevent crippling and disability in many cases if treatment begins early enough.

How Is RA Diagnosed?

RA can be notoriously difficult to diagnose, especially in its early stages. Its symptoms usually don't appear all at once, but typically reveal themselves slowly, over a period of months or years. Stiff, painful joints are usually among the first symptoms of RA, but they also occur in many other joint diseases. For this reason, diagnosing RA often requires ruling out other possible causes of the symptoms.

did you know

Women with RA often find that their disease abates during pregnancy—sometimes remarkably so. Unfortunately, the disease usually resumes its severity a month or two after delivery. And in some women RA appears for the first time in the weeks following childbirth. Whatever causes "pregnancy remissions" could help researchers develop new treatments for RA.

now and then

Doctors once believed that damage to a joint's bones didn't occur until many years after RA began affecting that joint. But recently, studies have shown that bone damage starts during the first year or two after RA's onset—pointing up the need for early diagnosis of RA and treatment to halt the inflammation that causes the damage.

The Four Degrees of RA

No two cases of RA proceed in exactly the same way. In fact, experts stress that RA's course in any patient is quite unpredictable. But they have identified four basic ways that the disease progresses—or, in some cases, doesn't.

1 In a few people—perhaps around 10 percent who develop it—RA is a temporary problem: These people experience a spontaneous and lasting remission that can't be attributed to any treatment they might be undergoing. When they happen, these spontaneous remissions usually occur within the first two years that people have RA. Another 10 percent of RA patients experience remissions, but the disease recurs later.

2 In the second type of RA, patients experience periodic flare-ups—weeks or months of painful, stiff, and swollen joints—that alternate with intervals of normal health. Their treatment will depend on whether their joints are damaged during the flare-ups and how well their joints function between flare-ups.

3 In the third type of RA, known as remitting-progressive, patients experience periodic flare-ups without returning to normal health between the attacks. Instead, during the periods between attacks, they have lingering joint inflammation that becomes increasingly more severe with each attack. If it isn't treated properly, remitting-progressive RA can eventually lead to significant joint damage.

4 The fourth type is called progressive RA, which is self-explanatory: The inflammation becomes more severe over time and causes gradually increasing pain, swelling, and—if severe inflammation lasts long enough—joint damage and disability.

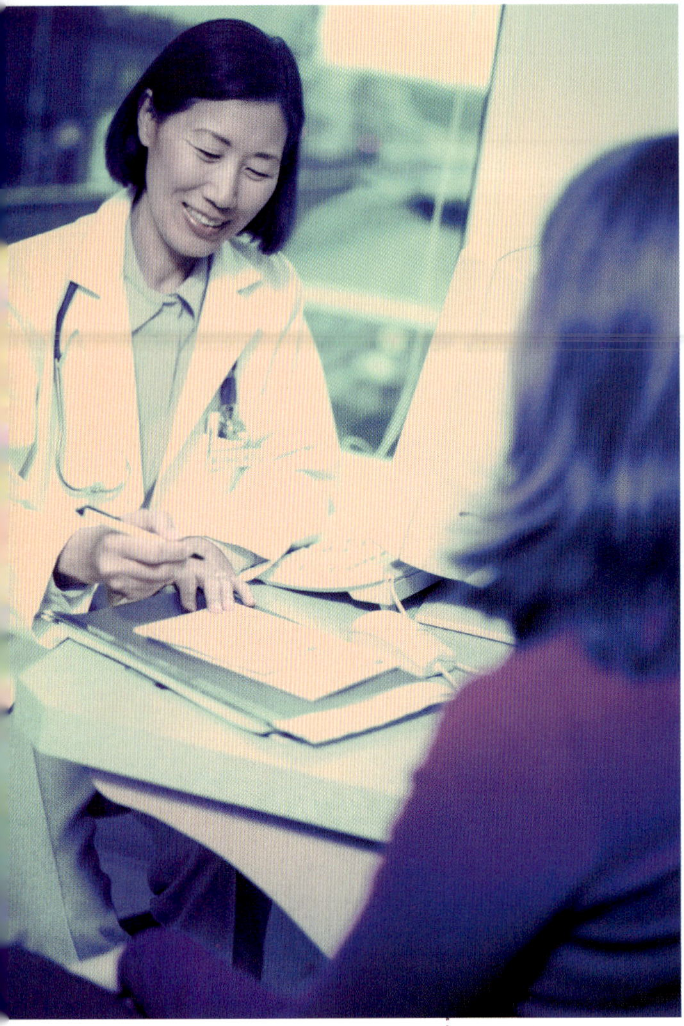

Medical history

As with OA, the first step is for a doctor to take your medical history (see page 48). The answers to certain questions—"Which joints are giving you trouble?", "Do the joints feel stiff in the morning and, if so, how long does the stiffness last?", "Are you experiencing a lot of fatigue?"—can help a doctor narrow the list of possible joint problems.

Physical exam

The doctor will focus on the affected joints, looking for the telltale signs of RA: joints that are tender, reddened, swollen, or warm, and have a limited range of motion. As noted earlier, problems in symmetrical joints—both elbows, for example—increase the odds that RA is present.

Lab test

Only one laboratory test is useful for confirming a diagnosis of RA: the rheumatoid factor test. Rheumatoid factor is an antibody produced by the synovial membranes of joints affected by RA and can be found in the blood of 80 to 90 percent of people with the condition. (Unfortunately, rheumatoid factor is often absent early in RA—when the test's help in diagnosing the disease is most needed.) In general, patients who test positive for rheumatoid factor tend to have more severe RA, and people with high levels of rheumatoid factor are more acutely affected than those with low amounts.

It's in the blood. Another test, the erythrocyte sedimentation rate, or "sed rate," is a broad indicator of inflammation in the body, including RA. Inflammation tends to make red blood cells sticky, so they form clumps that will settle ("sediment out") in a test tube. The greater the inflammation, the larger the red-cell clumps and the faster they'll fall to the bottom of the tube. This makes the sed rate useful for monitoring whether a treatment for RA is reducing inflammation. But because infections,

Rheumatic Rundown

Painful, swollen joints occur in a large number of joint ailments. Here is a rundown of rheumatic diseases with similar symptoms:

- Rheumatoid arthritis
- Ankylosing spondylitis
- Systemic lupus erythematosus
- Arthritis associated with psoriasis
- Reiter's syndrome
- Gout
- Pseudogout
- Bursitis

malignancies, and other problems can provoke inflammation, the sed rate is of limited help in diagnosing the condition.

An inside job. A useful but more invasive way to confirm that a person has some form of inflammatory arthritis is to evaluate synovial fluid removed from an affected joint by use of a needle. The fluid is examined under a microscrope to see if there are large numbers of neutrophils, white blood cells that gather at sites of inflammation.

X rays

These are of limited use in diagnosing RA. They often appear totally normal early in the course of the disease, even when symptoms are severe. In fact, X rays usually don't provide evidence of RA until significant and irreversible joint damage has occurred. At that point, X rays reveal that inflammation has destroyed cartilage and eroded the underlying bone.

What Now?

A diagnosis of RA can be sobering: The disease can cause significant joint damage and disability. It can disrupt people's lives, affecting their relationships and draining their financial resources. But you can blunt RA's impact if you approach the disease in the right way.

Don't panic. The great majority of people who are diagnosed with RA have relatively mild symptoms that can be controlled with proper treatment. Furthermore, breakthrough treatments for RA have been introduced in just the past few years, and even better treatments are expected in the near future.

what the studies show

In a large-scale study published in 1994, an average of nine months elapsed between the time RA patients first experienced symptoms and when they were finally diagnosed with RA.

Surviving Flare-Ups

For people diagnosed with any type of arthritis, "flare" becomes an important part of their vocabulary. Things may be going along smoothly—so smoothly you've almost forgotten you have arthritis—and then, suddenly, a flare.

Arthritis flares are times when things go bad: inflammation, pain, and stiffness resurface with a vengeance. Flares can be set off by many different things—overdoing things at the gym, lack of sleep, emotional stress.

Flares can severely challenge the patience—sometimes even the sanity—of people with arthritis. Successfully taking charge of arthritis means riding out a flare so that it causes the least amount of aggravation and despair.

Minimizing pain. The key is learning how to adjust to a flare without giving in to it. When a flare comes on, you'll want to give yourself more rest and protect the inflamed joints from further exertion. On the other hand, overprotecting a joint can be counterproductive, since long periods of inactivity can cause the muscles and tendons around a joint to weaken. You may also want to consult with your doctor about adjusting your medication in response to a flare.

Unfortunately, flares are an unvoidable part of arthritis. But knowing you can manage these periodic crises means you don't have to live in dread of them.

Tell your friends and family. Even people with mild cases of RA can expect to experience periodic "flares"—sudden worsenings of the inflammation that can temporarily disable a person with pain and fatigue. If family and friends are aware of this and other complications of RA, they'll be more understanding and more willing to pitch in to help when you're not feeling up to par.

Choosing the right doctor. If you've been diagnosed with RA, you owe it to yourself and your family to be treated by a rheumatologist, a physician who specializes in treating rheumatoid and other types of arthritis. More than most other diseases, RA demands close monitoring and fine-tuning of treatment to prevent permanent damage to joints. You need a doctor who is experienced in treating RA and who is familiar with the latest treatments.

Equally important, choose a doctor you feel comfortable with, since the two of you will have to work closely to develop an effective treatment plan.

Assemble a health-care team. In general, people with RA do best under the care of several health-care professionals. In addition to your physician, you may benefit from working with a physical therapist (who can help you set up an exercise program) and a psychologist or mental-health professional (who can steer you through the periods of depression and helplessness that RA patients may experience).

Set realistic goals. This is important for people with any type of arthritis but especially RA, a disease that can pose significant physical and emotional challenges. Setting and meeting realistic goals is vital to coping with the condition, and you can learn how to do that in this book.

Make use of resources. People with RA can benefit greatly from a wide variety of resources, including support groups and self-help courses sponsored by their local Arthritis Foundation chapter and support groups and health information offered on the Internet.

How Is RA Treated?

In RA, patient and doctor work together to achieve several goals:

- alleviate pain, stiffness, swelling, fatigue, and other symptoms
- reduce the inflammation
- slow down or halt the joint damage
- limit RA's interference with a patient's life

Drugs can put out the fire

Virtually all people diagnosed with RA must rely on drugs to control their disease. The arsenal of drugs falls generally into two classes: NSAIDs (nonsteroidal anti-inflammatory drugs) and

now and then

Until the late 1980s, doctors believed that early RA could be managed exclusively with NSAIDs and that disease-modifying anti-rheumatic drugs (DMARDs) weren't needed until joint damage showed up on X rays. They later realized that permanent joint damage can occur even in the first months of RA—despite the use of NSAIDs and long before damage can be seen on X rays. Now, experts agree that use of DMARDs should begin almost as soon as RA is diagnosed.

did you know

Recent studies suggest that fewer people are developing rheumatoid arthritis than in previous years, but no one knows the reason why.

Filtering Out RA

In March 1999 the FDA approved the Prosorba column, the first "nondrug alternative" for adults with moderate to severe RA who cannot tolerate DMARDs. During a two-hour process, the patient's blood is removed and passed through a machine that separates the plasma (liquid part of the blood) from the blood cells. The plasma is then passed through the Prosorba column, a device about the size of a coffee mug. The filtered plasma is then recombined with its blood cells, and the blood is reinfused into the patient.

The Prosorba treatment (carried out once a week for 12 weeks) can cause dramatic improvement in RA patients. Although researchers don't fully understand the column's mechanism of action, they believe it filters out proteins involved in the immune system's attack on the joints.

DMARDs (disease-modifying anti-rheumatic drugs). Successful treatment of RA usually requires taking both types.

NSAIDs for inflammation. NSAIDs are the mainstays of RA treatment. As their name implies, NSAIDs reduce inflammation and the symptoms it causes, including pain, stiffness, and swelling. The NSAIDs include ordinary aspirin, plus many other drugs such as diclofenac, ibuprofen, ketoprofen, naproxen, piroxicam, and sulindac. However, the high doses of NSAIDs used in treating RA can cause a nasty side effect: serious gastrointestinal bleeding.

Since 1998, the FDA has approved the first three of a new class of NSAIDs called COX-2 inhibitors. These drugs—Celebrex, Vioxx, and Mobic—relieve inflammation as well as standard NSAIDs while posing less risk for causing gastrointestinal problems. These COX-2 inhibitors are useful for people over 65, who are especially susceptible to bleeding from using standard NSAIDs.

Although NSAIDs counter inflammation, they don't prevent renegade synovial tissue from eroding cartilage and bone—the destructive process that inflammation sets in motion and that causes permanent joint damage.

DMARDs for joint damage. So-called disease-modifying anti-rheumatic drugs resemble NSAIDs in that they help to dampen RA's inflammation. But more important, the DMARDs can alter the course of RA by slowing down or halting the joint damage that can occur independently of inflammation. DMARDs are slow-acting drugs, and it may take several weeks before their effects are noticeable. People taking DMARDs must be closely monitored, because these drugs have the potential for causing serious adverse side effects.

For nearly 20 years, methotrexate—a drug first approved as a cancer treatment—has been the most widely prescribed DMARD. But three new DMARDs approved since 1998 have greatly enhanced the treatment of RA and have already transformed the lives of many people with the disease.

The next generation. Two of these new DMARDs—Enbrel (etanercept) and Remicade (infliximab) are genetically engineered drugs that neutralize tumor necrosis factor, a chemical that seems to play a major role in causing both inflammation and joint damage. Arava (leflunomide) is the third new DMARD and the only one that can be taken orally (all other DMARDs must be injected). Arava retards RA's progression by blocking an enzyme in white blood cells involved in the immune system's attack on the joints.

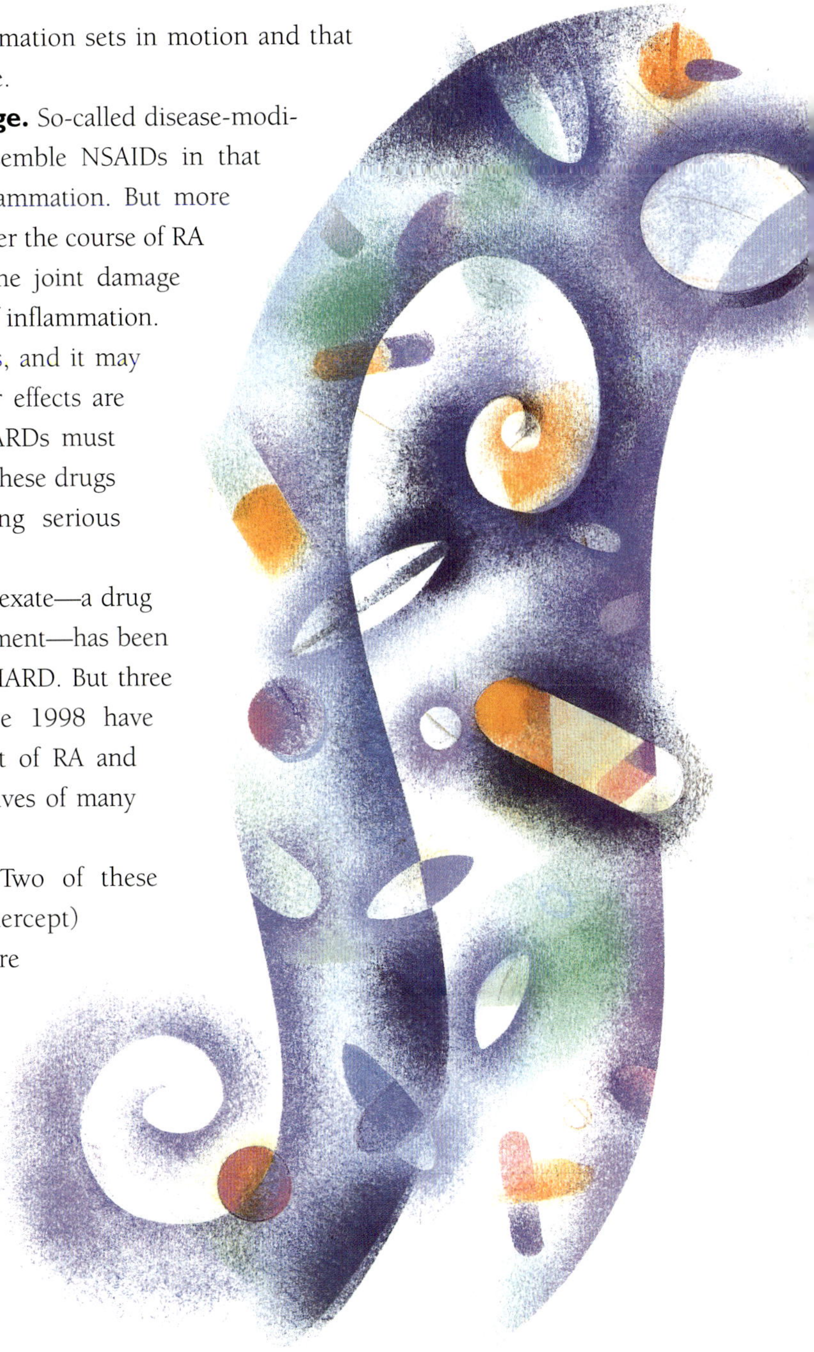

did you know

About 30 percent of FM patients in the U.S. have had to reduce their work hours or the amount of physical exertion they can put into their jobs. About 15 percent are disabled and receiving Social Security disability payments.

Surgery: A new lease on mobility

When RA's joint damage is severe, several types of surgical repair are possible. Total joint replacement with an artificial joint can dramatically improve pain and function in RA patients. Excellent results are now achieved in the replacement of knees, hips, and shoulders, but the outcome is less certain when elbows, wrists, and ankles are replaced.

Fibromyalgia: It's Not Just in Your Mind

If you literally ache all over, you may have fibromyalgia (FM)—one of the most vexing of all medical problems. One recent textbook described FM as a "chronic, poorly understood, and disabling condition." It is all of that and perhaps more.

FM is relatively common, affecting about five million Americans, or two percent of the general population. The overwhelming majority of FM patients—more than 75 percent—are women, and the ailment typically starts when a person is in her mid-40s. Fibromyalgia is a significant health problem, accounting for one of every six visits that people make to rheumatologists.

caution

Today, someone diagnosed with RA can expect to receive early and aggressive treatment with powerful drugs that can have serious side effects: all the more reason, experts say, to avoid a rush to diagnostic judgment. When the presence of RA is unclear, the best of all diagnostic tests is the test of time. It may take a few weeks or months of repeated assessment, but a "true" case of RA will eventually reveal itself.

What Is FM?

FM's main features are severe and widespread muscle pain that is most pronounced in the neck and shoulders, extreme fatigue, and—in most cases—poor sleep. Fibromyalgia can feel like a joint disease, but the pain actually occurs in nearby muscles, ligaments, and tendons.

FM's pain and other symptoms may persist for years—even for life—but may vary in intensity from day to day. Both inactivity and unaccustomed physical activity can make symptoms worse, and so can insomnia, humid weather, and emotional stress.

In addition to widespread persistent pain, fatigue, and poor sleep, people with FM typically report many other problems including:

- Irritable bowel syndrome (present in up to 50 percent of cases)
- Tension headache
- Problems concentrating or remembering
- Sense of swollen hands that are normal on examination
- Palpitations
- Depression

What Causes FM?

One of the most frustrating aspects of FM—for patients, their families, and their doctors—is the absence of any definite cause or causes. FM may well be the result of a complex interaction among many different physiological and psychological factors. For now, experts have proposed a number of theories for what causes FM, including:

Heredity/family

Research shows that FM patients are more likely than other people to have a family history of pain, depression, or alcoholism. Also, not surprisingly, FM is more common among relatives of FM patients than among relatives of nonaffected people.

The stress factor

Most researchers agree that stress is a key factor in FM. Studies show that FM patients report high levels of stress in their lives—more, for example, than in RA patients or in other people who don't have FM.

A recent study involving FM patients found that the greater their psychological distress, the more sensitive they are to pain and the more physical complaints they have. What's not clear is whether stress causes FM or is the consequence of living with a severe and sometimes disabling condition.

A real problem. Even if stress "causes" FM, the disorder clearly isn't "all in the mind," as some skeptics contend, but is a genuine medical problem. Mind-body research over the past decade shows that emotional stress can cause major changes in the body that adversely affect the nervous system, immune system, as well as hormone levels.

now and then

Until about 20 years ago FM was known as fibrositis, a condition of inflamed ("-itis") muscles, tendons, and other fibrous tissues. In 1979, Canadian physicians showed that fibrositis patients also suffered from extreme fatigue and, in almost all cases, problems with sleep. Studies also found that achy joints of fibrositis patients were not actually inflamed. So in 1981 Dr. Muhammad B. Yunus, professor of medicine at the University of Illinois College of Medicine at Peoria, proposed the term "fibromyalgia," which roughly means achy muscles and other soft tissues. The American Medical Association recognized FM as a medical disorder in 1987.

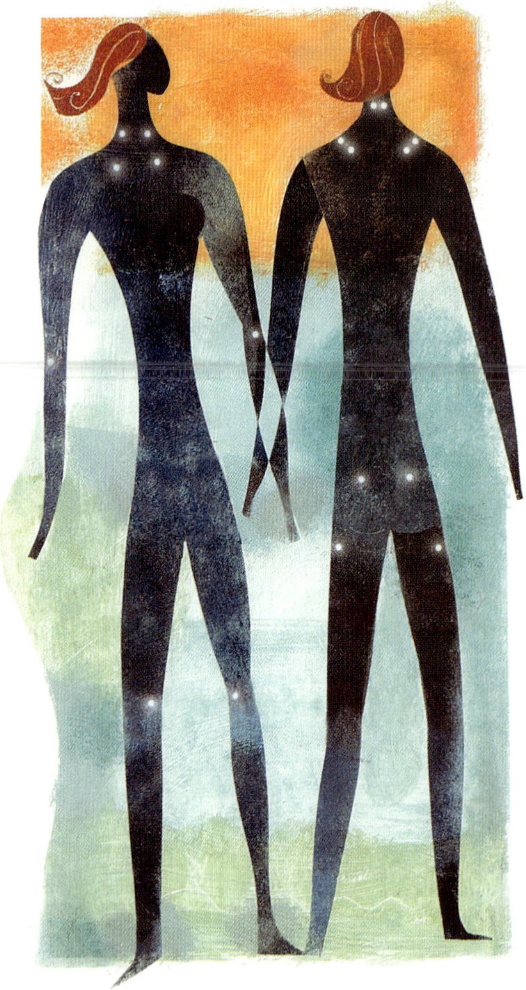

High levels of substance P

Responsible for alerting the nervous system to a painful injury of the tissues, this chemical is found at elevated levels in the cerebrospinal fluid of people with FM. In some people with FM, levels of substance P consistently measure two to three times above normal; in others, substance P levels gradually increase as symptoms become more severe. Increased substance P levels, perhaps induced by stress, may help explain the recent finding that FM patients have lower pain thresholds—greater sensitivity to painful stimuli—than people who don't have the condition.

Injuries, accidents, or traumas

Some people can trace the onset of their FM to relatively minor accidents such as fender-bender collisions. But most experts doubt that minor trauma can produce the long-lasting effects on muscles and other soft tissue throughout the body that characterizes FM.

Tendering a Diagnosis of FM

The 18 tender points are nine paired points (the insides of both elbows, for example) on the front and back of the body between the knees and the neck (see above). Pressing the tender points firmly will hurt anyone; but in someone with FM, pressing tender points lightly—with just enough pressure to cause the fingernail to blanch—can cause excruciating pain.

A diagnosis of fibromyalgia requires pain in at least 11 of these tender points. But as a practical matter, experts believe that someone with long-standing musculoskeletal pain, plus impaired sleep that doesn't relieve fatigue, can still be diagnosed with FM even if fewer than 11 tender points are painful to the touch.

Taking Charge of Fibromyalgia

Sometimes it's easier to have a clear-cut medical problem than one like FM, with its largely subjective symptoms of pain and fatigue. People with FM must often contend with skeptical doctors and family members who doubt whether their complaints are real.

Hands-on benefits. For this and other reasons—including a lack of truly effective treatments—FM can be an especially difficult illness to cope with, but also one that can be greatly helped by the take-charge approach espoused in this book. Studies consistently show that by gaining self-empowerment—believing in your ability to control your disease and overcome symptoms—FM patients can improve their mood, decrease pain, and better tolerate the pain they still have.

How Is FM Diagnosed?

A striking feature of FM is that standard diagnostic tests—blood chemistries or X rays, for example—appear perfectly normal. As a result, a diagnosis of FM must be made by clinical examination. In 1990, after comparing FM patients with control patients, the American College of Rheumatology set out specific criteria for physicians to use in diagnosing FM. To be diagnosed with FM, patients must have:

- widespread muscle pain that has been present for at least three months
- pain in at least 11 of 18 "tender points" when a doctor pushes on those spots

BONING UP: Next to osteoarthritis, FM is the second most commonly diagnosed musculoskeletal disorder.

What Now?

If you're like many people, you may actually be relieved to receive a diagnosis of FM: Some people spend years seeking an explanation for their symptoms, with numerous doctors telling them that the problem is all in their head.

Accentuate the positive. The upside for people with FM is that it doesn't involve damage to the joints. Even though you may hurt all over and feel exhausted, you won't be crippled by FM. On the other hand, FM tends to linger—sometimes for life—although the severity of the pain and fatigue may ebb and flow over the years. One of the keys to coping with FM is overcoming the sleep disturbances that contribute to FM's sometimes disabling fatigue.

How Is FM Treated?

Since there is no known cause for FM, treatment is aimed at easing its symptoms—not an easy task. For example, drugs that work well at relieving pain associated with many types of arthritic problems—ibuprofen and other NSAIDs—are notably ineffective against the pain of fibromyalgia. This difficulty in finding effective treatments often only adds to the frustration that many FM patients experience.

Exercise. Although no single treatment has proven universally effective against FM, physicians who have cared for

Fibromyalgia Strategy Guide: What Else You Can Do

- Eat several small meals during the day to maintain a steady supply of protein and carbohydrate for proper muscle function.
- Take hot baths or showers—especially in the morning—to soothe soreness, increase circulation, and relieve stiffness.
- Find a massage therapist familiar with fibromyalgia. A technique called trigger-point therapy can be extremely helpful in reducing pain.
- Cut back on caffeine, alcohol, and sugar, which often cause fatigue.
- Get at least eight hours of sleep a night.

many FM patients seem to agree that aerobic exercise should be a part of any treatment program. For one thing, aerobic exercise improves sleep—almost always poor among FM patients—and better sleep helps relieve FM's extreme fatigue. In addition, studies show that aerobic exercise helps to ease muscle pain and tenderness in FM patients.

Many fibromyalgia patients find that a combination of different treatments is the best route to relief for their symptoms. Other possible treatments for FM include:

caution

FM patients embarking on an exercise regimen should start out slowly, especially if they've been inactive, since unaccustomed exertion can cause severe pain. You should also avoid high-impact exercises—jogging or tennis, for example—and opt for biking, walking, or swimming instead.

Low doses of antidepressants. These drugs—tricyclics like amitriptyline and SSRIs like Prozac—are given mainly to improve sleep and relax muscles rather than to relieve depression. Both types of drugs seem to have physiological effects on the nervous system that may explain the improvement in fatigue and nonrejuvenating sleep experienced by people with FM. In general, drugs that improve sleep have proven to be the most useful medications for treating fibromyalgia.

BONING UP: Some studies suggest that combinations of magnesium and malic acid, L-carnitine, and co-enzyme Q-10, when taken with a high-potency multivitamin/antioxidant combination, may help FM patients.

NSAIDs. These painkilling drugs have generally proven disappointing in clinical studies involving FM patients. But some people with FM may benefit from using them.

Topical treatments. Applying creams containing the ingredient capsaicin—a substance derived from chili peppers—to painful areas seems to help some people with fibromyalgia.

Acupuncture. This ancient treatment has shown promise in treating several types of musculoskeletal problems, including FM.

what the studies show

In one study, published in 1992 in the *British Medical Journal*, 70 FM patients were randomly assigned to receive six treatments using either electroacupuncture (electric current is applied to the needles) or superficial "needling." At the end of the treatment period, patients receiving genuine acupuncture treatment were experiencing significantly less pain than patients receiving the sham treatment.

Ankylosing Spondylitis: Back Pain with a Twist

Anywhere from 500,000 to two million Americans are believed to suffer from AS, a chronic inflammation of the spine. It is three times more common in men than in women, but recent research suggests that the ratio may be much more equal: women often have much milder cases that usually escape detection.

AS is mainly a disease of young people, often beginning before age 20 and rarely affecting people over 40. Once thought to be part of rheumatoid arthritis, we now know that it is related but separate.

What Is AS?

AS is a type of chronic arthritis that mainly affects the spine. (*Ankylosing* means stiff, *spondyl* refers to the spine, and *itis* means inflammation.) In AS, the inflammation occurs in joints and in areas where tendons and ligaments attach to bones. In severe cases, inflammation of the spine can actually cause the spinal vertebrae to fuse.

Older people who walk hunched over and looking down at the ground are usually in the late stages of AS. The good news is that today's treatment approaches can almost always prevent AS from becoming a disabling or crippling condition.

What Causes AS?

As with many types of arthritis, the cause of AS is not known. But genes have a strong influence, since AS occurs primarily in people who have a genetic marker, or protein, called HLA-B27 on the surface of white blood cells. Someone who carries the HLA-B27 gene has a one to two percent risk of developing AS—but the risk can rise to 20 percent if a first-degree relative (parent or sibling) has the disease.

How Does AS Progress?

AS typically begins gradually, almost insidiously. The first symptoms are usually aches and pains in the lower back caused by inflammation of the sacroiliac joints, located in the lower back on both sides of the spine and just above the buttocks. (Lower back pain that begins gradually and persists for months is often a tipoff for the disease.) The backache can be quite severe, interfering with sleep and causing a person to roll sideways to avoid bending the back when getting out of bed.

BONING UP: One way to distinguish between a ruptured disk and early ankylosing spondylitis is that while disk pain is improved with rest, the pain of AS usually gets worse with rest and better with movement.

Ascending pain. As it progresses, AS and its inflammation may move to the upper back and may also spread to other joints as well, especially the neck, hips, and shoulders. The spine becomes stiff due to pain and muscle spasms. In the final stages of AS, chronic inflammation can cause bony bridges to form between the vertebrae, resulting in the spine fusing permanently into a bent and inflexible position.

AS is a systemic disease, so it sometimes affects areas of the body beyond the joints. People with AS may experience fatigue, weight loss, poor appetite, and—in about 25 percent of patients—an inflammatory eye condition known as iritis, which causes redness and tearing. People with severe and long-standing AS may experience damage to heart tissue that requires the implantation of a pacemaker.

How Is AS Diagnosed?

Ankylosing spondylitis can be a challenging disease to diagnose, especially in its early stages. In general, the medical history alone can offer a doctor several clues that, when pieced together, point to a diagnosis of AS:

did you know

Ankylosing spondylitis can be traced to antiquity. In 1912, archaeologists unearthed an Egyptian mummy from about 3000 B.C. The mummy's spine was described as "a rigid block of stone" extending from its base to the neck.

- The patient is a male between 16 and 35
- Back pain and stiffness developed gradually
- Symptoms have been present continually for more than three months
- The patient has back stiffness on waking up in the morning
- Exercise helps to relieve the stiffness and pain

The physical exam

The doctor will assess the flexibility of a patient's spine—asking him to bend over to touch his toes, for example. The doctor may also press on the patient's sacroiliac joints to see if they are tender and measure his lung function to see if the patient has trouble inhaling completely.

Lab tests

Testing the patient's blood for the presence of the HLA-B27 marker can help confirm a diagnosis of AS or help rule out similar diseases like rheumatoid arthritis or lupus. But otherwise, diagnostic tests are not very useful in AS.

X rays

These can provide a definitive diagnosis of AS, but signs of the disease usually don't show up on an X ray until about five years after the disease begins. The first joints to shown signs of ankylosing spondylitis are usually the sacroiliac joints, which appear fuzzy on X rays because their surfaces have been eroded by inflammation.

BONING UP: Tenderness where a tendon attaches to a bone—a sharp pain in the shoulders, buttocks, back of the knees, or the heel—can be a sign of early-stage ankylosing spondylitis.

what the studies show

In studies of people with AS, the disease leveled off in almost all of them, but as many as 40 percent had restricted joint motion of the spine. Also, in the vast majority of AS sufferers, breathing ability was impaired.

What Now?

Someone recently diagnosed with AS should feel reasonably upbeat. Chances are you've been diagnosed early in the course of the disease. Today's treatments—primarily exercise and the use of NSAIDs—can almost always prevent AS from progressing to the point of irreversible spinal rigidity. These treatments also do a good job of alleviating pain and stiffness and enable most people with ankylosing spondylitis to remain active and lead normal, fulfilling lives.

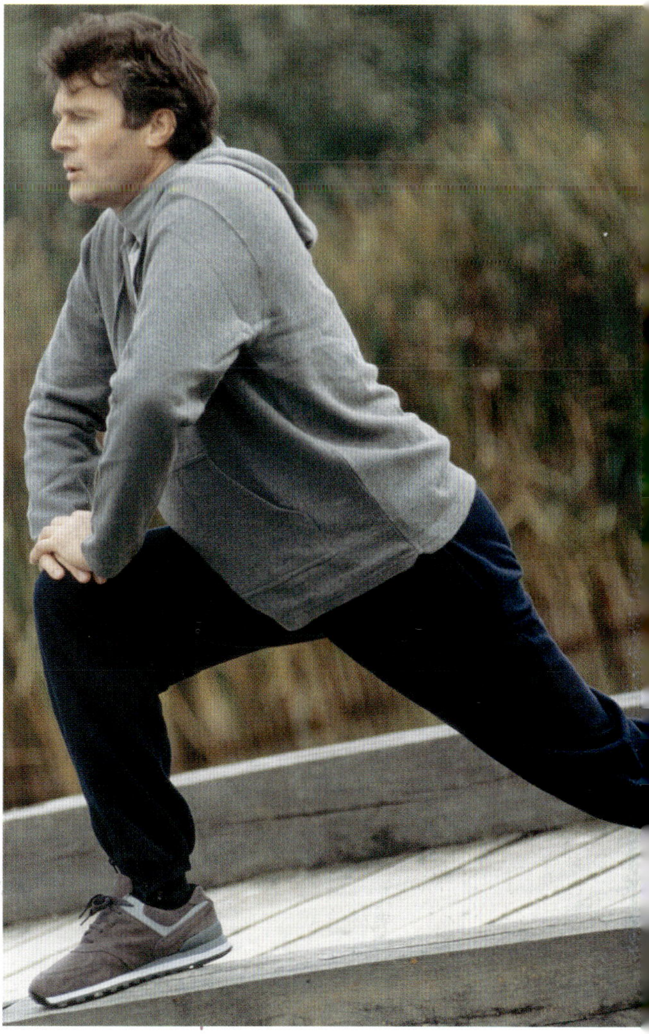

How Is AS Treated?

Today's treatments allow most people with AS to lead normal lives, but a take-charge approach emphasizing exercise is absolutely essential for success.

The healing power of exercise. Regular activity enables AS patients to maintain a limber spine and prevent spinal deformity. Daily stretching exercises for the spine are especially recommended. Swimming may be the best overall exercise for AS patients, since it stretches the back but doesn't stress it the way running or other weight-bearing exercises do. Patients suffering from AS must also maintain as straight a spine as possible, by practicing good posture when sitting or standing and by sleeping on a firm mattress.

Drug therapy. Regular use of NSAIDs is also important in treating AS—mainly because of its effect on exercise. These anti-inflammatory drugs ease pain and stiffness enough to allow patients to engage in an active exercise program, which is critical to preventing the disease from worsening.

Systemic Lupus Erythematosus: The Great Impostor

Lupus is a chronic disease that usually inflames the joints—and also affects the skin, kidneys, blood vessels, nervous system, and virtually every other

did you know

Before corticosteroids were available, the mortality rate was high for lupus. Most people with serious kidney disease died and those without renal disease survived in only 50 percent of the cases.

People with lupus may want to avoid alfalfa in any form—including sprouts, seeds, tablets, and tea. It contains a substance called canavanine, which some experts think triggers flare-ups.

organ in the body. About one in 2,000 people develop lupus, which is mainly a disease of young women. In fact, women are afflicted with lupus about five times more often than men.

What Is Lupus?

Lupus is an autoimmune disease in which the immune system produces large numbers of several different types of antibodies that attack the body's own tissues, causing symptoms that strongly resemble those of rheumatoid arthritis.

What Causes Lupus?

Experts believe people inherit a susceptibility to lupus: It is known to affect identical twins, and first-degree relatives of patients are much more likely than other people to develop the disease. In lupus, the body makes antibodies that attack the nuclei and other components of its own cells.

BONING UP: Discoid lupus is limited only to the skin. Symptoms include a rash on the face, neck, and scalp. This type of lupus does not affect internal organs.

Some triggering event, such as an infection or stress, may provoke lupus in genetically susceptible people. Since lupus is almost always a disease that strikes young women, hormones may also play a role in causing it.

Drug-induced lupus. Interestingly, many drugs commonly used to treat other diseases can cause "temporary" lupus, which disappears when the drug is stopped. Hydralazine (a high-blood-pressure medication), procainamide (used to treat irregular heartbeats), and isoniazid (a tuberculosis drug) are the chief culprits. This finding has attracted the attention of researchers who are studying how the drugs alter the immune system—findings that could shed light on how lupus develops and lead to better treatments.

How Does Lupus Progress?

Typically, a young woman will develop an array of symptoms over several months that may include worsening fatigue, weight loss, a mild fever, and a great deal of joint pain that doesn't involve swelling or joint tenderness. About half of people with early lupus will also develop a butterfly-shaped facial rash that people once thought resembled a wolf's face—hence the name *lupus* (Latin for wolf). This distinctive rash can help in diagnosis.

Later in the course of the disease, other parts of the body may become affected, including the gastrointestinal tract (nausea, abdominal pain), blood cells (anemia), tissue surrounding the heart and lungs (inflammation), and the nervous system (headaches, seizures, strokes, and hallucinations). The kidneys are an especially important target, and damage to the organs can lead to kidney failure in late-stage lupus.

Other health problems that may occur in the later stages of lupus include cognitive problems such as decreased memory and difficulty doing simple math calculations. In addition, deaths from heart attack can occur due to atherosclerosis.

How Is Lupus Diagnosed?

Since it can affect so many parts of the body, lupus can mimic many diseases—making diagnosis very difficult, especially in the early stages of the condition. Presence of the butterfly rash can

Growing a New Immune System

Tulane University Medical Center in New Orleans is performing an experimental treatment for severe lupus sufferers: bone marrow transplantation. Stem cells—from which all other blood cells evolve—are harvested from a person with lupus. The person is then treated with chemotherapy and radiation therapy to destroy his or her defective immune system. Afterward, the stem cells are put back into the person intravenously where new, healthy blood cells begin to form. It is hoped that the patient will grow a new immune system. Northwestern Memorial Hospital in Chicago is also using stem-cell transplantation to treat lupus.

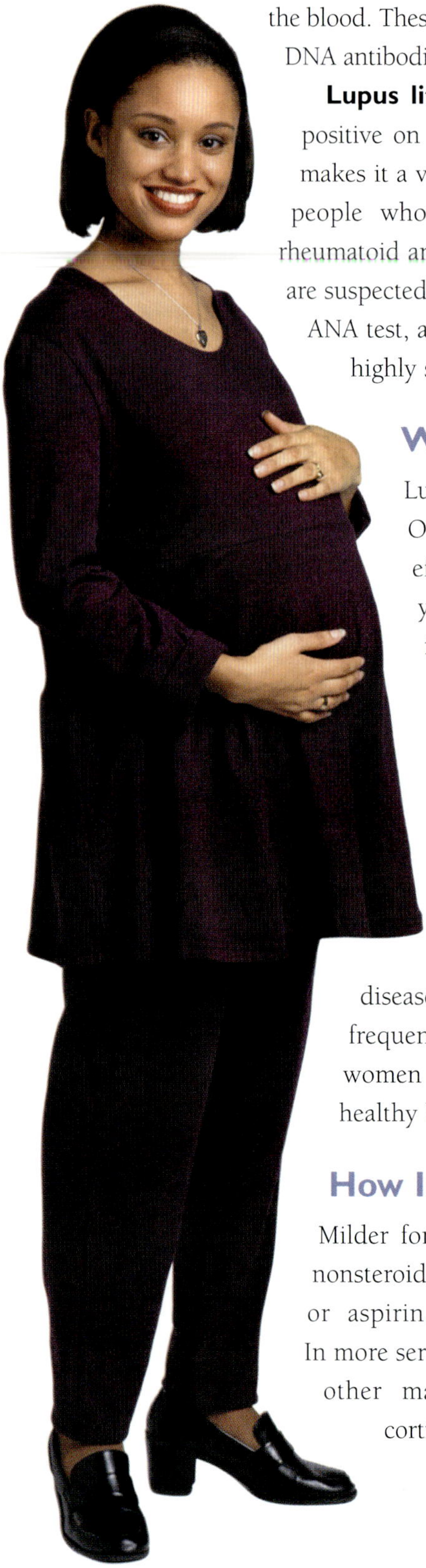

certainly help a doctor make the diagnosis, but a definitive diagnosis sometimes depends on two tests that detect antibodies in the blood. These antibodies—anti-nuclear antibodies and anti-DNA antibodies—both attack the nucleus of a patient's cells.

Lupus litmus tests. Virtually all lupus patients test positive on the anti-nuclear antibody (ANA) test, which makes it a very good screening test for the condition. But people who have other types of arthritis, including rheumatoid arthritis, can also test positive. So patients who are suspected of having lupus, and who test positive on the ANA test, are given the anti-DNA antibody test, which is highly specific for the condition.

What Now?

Lupus can certainly be a very serious disease. On the plus side, most people with lupus can be effectively treated. Especially over the past 30 years, treatment for lupus has dramatically improved, and some of the worst complications—such as kidney failure—can now almost always be avoided.

Lupus and fertility. Most people diagnosed with lupus are young women, and many are concerned that the condition may impair their ability to have children. Here again the news is largely reassuring: In women severely affected by lupus, the disease may indeed impair fertility and cause more frequent miscarriages. But the great majority of women with lupus can become pregnant and have healthy babies.

How Is Lupus Treated?

Milder forms of lupus can usually be managed with nonsteroidal anti-inflammatory drugs such as ibuprofen or aspirin, which reduce inflammation and pain. In more serious cases, when lupus affects the kidneys or other major organs, patients are usually given corticosteroids—potent anti-inflammatory drugs that can also cause serious side effects. Some two thirds of lupus patients are treated with corticosteroids.

In the most severe lupus cases, patients are treated with immunosuppressants—powerful drugs used to prevent a transplant recipient from rejecting a donated organ. They work similarly in lupus patients, by suppressing the immune system's attack on the body's organs.

Other Types of Arthritis: In a Nutshell

Below and on the next couple of pages you will find only a small number of the types of arthritis you may be suffering from. Don't use these nutshell descriptions as a way of diagnosing your aches and pains. Make an appointment with your physician and undergo a thorough physical. Your symptoms are unique and only your doctor can determine what you may have.

Finding the appropriate specialist or specialists is an important part of diagnosing your symptoms. It may take time to rule out the many other disorders that mimic your particular manifestation of arthritis before your doctor can make a final diagnosis. Once again, you and your doctor should be the architects of this important diagnosis process.

Reiter's Syndrome: It Starts with an Infection

Reiter's syndrome is a chronic, intermittent, inflammatory condition that affects not only the joints (usually starting in the knees, feet, or ankles) but also other parts of the body as well, particularly the urethra and the eyes, which can develop conjunctivitis. The syndrome is most common in men ages 20 to 40, who develop it after becoming infected with a sexually transmitted disease, and also occurs in people with a genetic susceptibility traceable to the HLA-B27 gene.

what the studies show

New studies show that microbes commonly cause rheumatoid arthritis and other rheumatic diseases in chimpanzees, rats, swine, poultry, and other domestic animals. The two culprits are mycoplasmas and Chlamydia—parasitic bacteria that produce Reiter's syndrome in the connective tissue of genetically susceptible people.

BONING UP: Reiter's syndrome is called a reactive arthritis because the joint inflammation appears to be a reaction to an infection originating in an area other than the joints.

Causes and symptoms. The condition is caused by the body's abnormal response to infections (either sexually transmitted diseases or infections of the gastrointestinal tract). Symptoms include inflammation of the urethra, conjunctivitis, and joint pain and inflammation—usually of the knees and toes and areas where tendons are attached to bones, such as the heels.

The combination of joint, genital, urinary, skin, and eye symptoms leads a doctor to suspect Reiter's syndrome. Because these symptoms may not appear simultaneously, the disease may not be diagnosed for several months. No simple laboratory tests are available to confirm the diagnosis.

What can be done. Antibiotics are used to treat the infection and NSAIDs can minimize pain and inflammation in the joint. Although the patient often recovers, the arthritic symptoms may continue on and off for many years.

what the studies show

One study showed that eating fresh or canned cherries (eight ounces a day) may help keep gout at bay by reducing levels of uric acid. Strawberries, blueberries, celery, or celery seed extract may have a similar beneficial effect.

Gout: The Arthritis of Kings

Gout attacks occur when excess levels of uric acid in the blood form needle-like crystals that typically settle in one of the joints—most commonly in the big toe but sometimes in the knee or knuckles. Once in the joint, these abrasive particles can cause excruciating pain and inflammation. The condition has afflicted royalty and the well-to-do through the ages.

Causes and symptoms. It's uncertain what precipitates a gout attack, though some factors may put you at risk. A quarter of those who suffer from gout have a family history of the illness, and three-quarters have high triglyceride levels. Men who gain a lot of weight between ages 20 and 40 are particularly vulnerable. Excessive alcohol intake, high blood pressure, kidney disease, exposure to lead, crash diets, and certain medications (including antibiotics, diuretics, and cancer chemotherapy drugs) may also play a role. For some people, eating foods high in chemicals called purines (such as liver or anchovies) can cause flare-ups.

Gout is diagnosed by identifying uric acid crystals in synovial fluid, usually by removing fluid from the joint through a needle. X rays can be helpful and may reveal uric acid deposits and bone damage if you have suffered from repeated inflammations.

Boning Up: Drinking plenty of water, up to two quarts a day, helps to increase the excretion of uric acid.

What can be done. Avoiding purine-rich foods (liver and anchovies, seafoods, dried peas and beans) can help prevent gout attacks. Keeping your weight down can also help, as does avoiding foods that are high in fat and refined carbohydrates. The biggest treatment advance in managing gout is drugs—allopurinol, probenecide, and sulfinpyrazone—that prevent gout attacks by controlling uric acid levels in the blood. The drug colchicine, derived from the autumn crocus, is one of the oldest known remedies for gout. But a newer injectable form of the drug appears to work quickly and without side effects.

Pseudogout: Condition of the Aged

This condition is very similar to gout but is caused by different types of crystals—in this case, calcium pryophosphate dihydrate crystals, which typically form for no reason. Pseudogout is common among older people, affecting about three percent of people in their 60s and as many as half of all people over 90.

Causes and symptoms. Although the cause of pseudogout is unknown, it may occur in people who have an abnormally high calcium level in the blood, an abnormally high iron level in the tissues, or abnormally low blood levels of magnesium. Symptoms vary widely. Some people have attacks of painful arthritis, usually in the knees, wrists, or other relatively large joints. Other people have lingering, chronic pain and stiffness in joints of the arms and legs, which doctors may confuse with rheumatoid arthritis. Pseudogout is diagnosed in the same manner as gout—removing fluid from the joint through a needle.

did you know

Although between 10 percent and 20 percent of Americans have high uric acid levels, only a small percentage of them ever actually develop gout.

What can be done. NSAIDs are used to reduce pain and inflammation and colchicine may be given intravenously to relieve the inflammation and pain during attacks.

Polymyositis: Attack of the Muscles

Polymyositis is a chronic connective tissue disease characterized by painful inflammation and degeneration of the muscles. The condition occurs in adults from ages 40 to 60 or in children ages 5 to 15 years. Women are twice as likely as men to develop the condition.

Causes and symptoms. Although the cause is unknown, viruses or autoimmune reactions may play a role. Cancer may also trigger the disease. Symptoms, which may begin during or just after an infection, include muscle weakness (particularly in the upper arms, hips, and thighs), muscle and joint pain, a rash, difficulty in swallowing, a fever, fatigue, and weight loss.

Polymyositis is often diagnosed by measuring muscle weakness at the shoulders or hips, or detecting a characteristic rash or increased blood levels of certain muscle enzymes.

What can be done. Restricting activities when the inflammation is most intense often helps. Generally, a corticosteroid (usually prednisone), taken orally, slowly improves strength and relieves pain and swelling, controlling the disease. In some cases, though, prednisone actually worsens the disease. In these cases, immunosuppressive drugs are used instead of, or in addition to, prednisone.

what the studies show

Recent studies suggest that a form of vitamin D may help psoriatic patients.

Psoriatic Arthritis: From Skin to Joints

Psoriatic arthritis resembles rheumatoid arthritis, but doesn't produce the antibodies characteristic of RA. A negative rheumatoid factor test helps distinguish it from rheumatoid arthritis. It affects about 10 percent of people who have the skin disease psoriasis. Psoriatic arthritis may develop at any age, but typically between the ages of 30 and 50, with heredity appearing to play a significant role in susceptibility.

Causes and symptoms. Psoriasis (a skin condition causing flare-ups of red, scaly rashes and thickened, pitted nails) may precede or follow the joint inflammation. Psoriatic arthritis usually affects joints of the fingers and toes. The joints may become swollen and deformed when inflammation is chronic.

What can be done. Treatment is aimed at controlling the skin rash and alleviating the joint inflammation. Several drugs that are effective in treating rheumatoid arthritis are also used to treat psoriatic arthritis. They include gold compounds, methotrexate, cyclosporine, and sulfasalazine. Another drug, etretinate, is usually effective in severe cases, but its side effects may be serious.

Lyme Arthritis: The Biting Truth

Lyme disease is now considered a trigger for rheumatoid arthritis. The most common tick-borne disease in the U.S., Lyme disease most commonly occurs on the East Coast from Virginia to Massachusetts, in Wisconsin and Minnesota, and parts of Northern California and the Pacific Northwest.

Causes and symptoms. People become infected when bitten by deer ticks that carry Lyme bacteria (known as *Borrellia burgdoferi*). Early Lyme disease symptoms include a ring-like rash at the point of initial infection and flu-like symptoms such as fatigue, fever, chills, and headache. If you are suffering the general symptoms listed above and have recently been in a Lyme hot zone, it's advisable to request a blood test that specifically looks for Lyme disease.

Prompt treatment with antibiotics can cure the infection. But without treatment, about 50 percent of infected people experience intermittent arthritis in various joints. The arthritis usually clears up on its own, but about 10 percent of people develop chronic inflammatory arthritis, most often in the knee.

What can be done. The best strategy is to avoid tick bites. People who go outside in Lyme-disease areas should wear light-colored clothes (so ticks will be visible), tuck pant cuffs into socks (to keep ticks away from the skin), use repellents containing the ingredient DEET, and conduct daily "tick checks" to remove ticks before they can bite. A vaccine against Lyme received marketing approval in 1998. Known as LYMErix, the vaccine protects about 80 percent of people and is given in three doses costing a total of about $150 (not including doctor's fees).

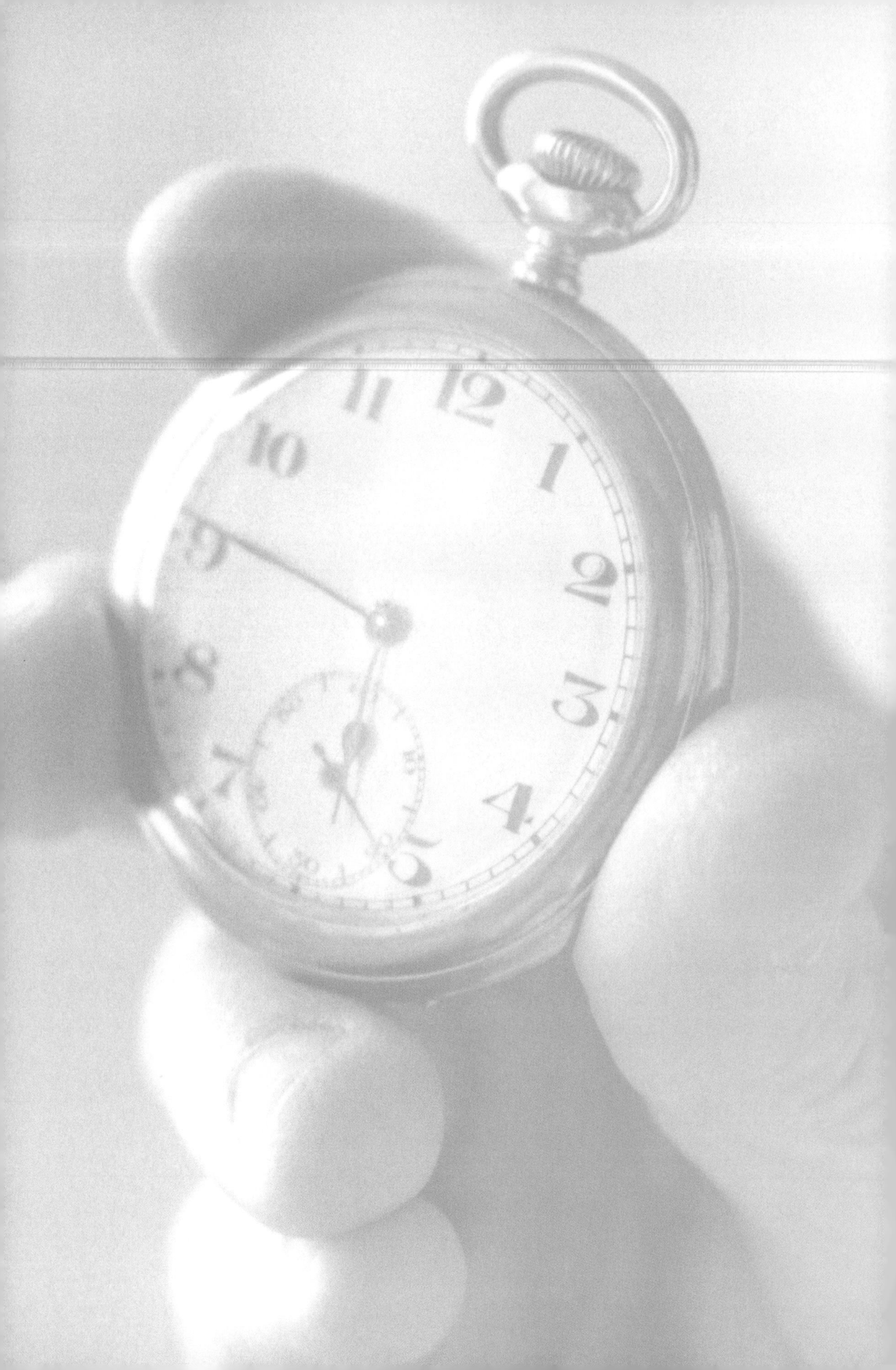

3 Taking Charge Now

As you take charge of your arthritis, you will be participating in the self-empowerment movement. This powerful approach will not only help you manage your condition but also sidestep the depression and hopelessness that often afflict arthritis patients.

KEY CONCEPT

The take-charge approach puts "the patient" back into "patient care." It helps people develop confidence in their ability to control and surmount even very severe arthritis symptoms.

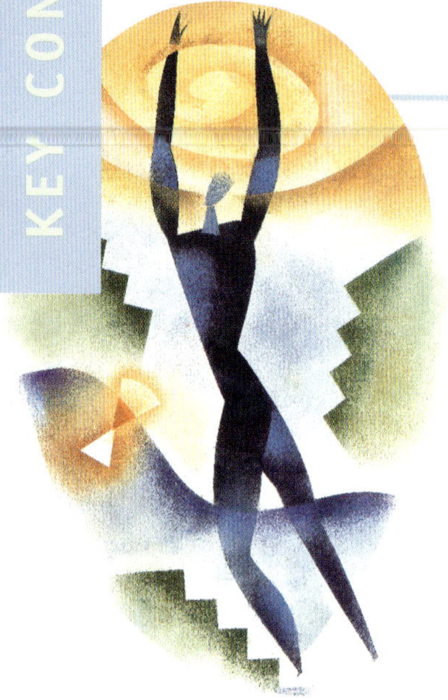

The Chronic Question: What Works for Arthritis

Acute and chronic health problems are very different. Acute health problems appear abruptly and don't last long: They typically either get better on their own (food poisoning, colds, or bruises, for example) or respond promptly to treatment (surgery to remove an inflamed appendix, penicillin to kill bacteria responsible for causing strep throat).

Arthritis and other chronic illnesses usually develop slowly and then linger—"chronic," by definition, means you have a problem indefinitely or even for life. And although acute health problems usually run a predictable course of illness followed by healing and cure, a diagnosis of arthritis involves much more uncertainty and many more questions:

- Will I have to give up my favorite activities?
- Can therapies keep my disease from progressing or help stabilize it?
- Will my pain and disability worsen?
- Will additional joints become affected?
- Can I continue to provide for my family?
- Can I perform the simple activities of everyday life that allow me to stay independent?

- How can I deal with the anger and frustration I feel?
- How will this affect my relationships with family and friends?

Boning Up: Always use the strongest and largest joints and muscles for the job. Getting up from a chair can place a great deal of strain on your hands if you push yourself with your fingertips. Instead of using your fingers or knuckles, use your palms to help you achieve liftoff.

Patient in Charge

All people with chronic health problems must deal with complex challenges every day. Even as they cope with their condition medically and surgically, they face tremendous uncertainty regarding the course of their disease and its impact on their lives. Add all these burdens to the pain and disability caused by the chronic illness itself, and patients can become frustrated and depressed.

Clearly, the key ingredient in managing a chronic condition is the patient's own involvement in making the decisions about his or her care.

Passive to aggressive. This need for patients to participate in their own health care may seem obvious now. But until recently, most patients with chronic health problems took a passive approach to treatment. They went to the doctor to find out how they were doing and rarely asked questions. If a drug wasn't helping or was causing stomach pain or some other adverse effect, they would rarely complain: After all, who were they to question the doctor's wisdom or to judge whether a treatment was working?

"Because of its chronic nature, arthritis patients must learn to manage and cope with the disease on a day-to-day basis. Their ability to succeed in this task commonly differentiates those who are incapacitated from those who continue to lead full and active lives...."

—Kate Lorig and Halsted Holman, arthritis self-management studies

Accentuate the Positive

You are probably familiar with Norman Vincent Peale's book, *The Power of Positive Thinking*. The take-charge approach to arthritis emphasizes something similar: the power of a positive attitude. When people adopt a take-charge attitude toward their arthritis, studies have shown that the new attitude itself can do wonders for their pain and disability.

Stay the course. This approach was emphasized in the Arthritis Self-Management Program developed by Stanford University in 1979. The Arthritis Foundation adopted the program in 1984 for its arthritis self-help course, offered through local Arthritis Foundation affiliates nationwide. Between 8,000 and 12,000 American adults enroll in the course every year, attending a weekly two-hour class for six weeks.

The program is also used in other countries, including Canada and Australia. So far, more than 300,000 people with arthritis have gone through the self-management program since it was developed.

Numerous studies have evaluated the success of self-management courses in improving the health of arthritis patients. In doing their follow-up studies, researchers had expected that the behaviors taught in the course—exercising more and eating healthier, for example—would have the biggest impact on improving participants' health. But the experts made a surprising finding.

Learned optimism. Participants had indeed changed their behavior for the better after taking the course, and they experienced significantly less pain and disability compared with patients who hadn't enrolled. But their improved health did not flow primarily from the behavior changes they'd made. Instead, the researchers found, participants' success in regaining their health hinged mainly on something else they got from the course: the confidence that they were able to control their arthritis symptoms.

A take-charge attitude, it turns out, can be learned—and is the key ingredient for overcoming arthritis.

what the studies show

People who take arthritis self-help courses not only reduce pain but also save money. A 1998 study calculated that, over a four-year period, the pain relief achieved by participants translates into a cost savings of $320 per person and a cost savings for the health-care system of $267 per person. The cost savings result mainly from a need for fewer doctor visits.

The Course That Changes Lives

In follow-up studies involving people enrolled in arthritis self-management courses, researchers found that the positive attitude gained by participants is crucial for reducing pain and disability. The studies also produced a number of other intriguing results, including:

1 Twenty months after completing the course, participants on average had reduced their pain by 20 percent, their depression by 14 percent, and visits to physicians by 35 percent compared with their situation before enrolling.

2 The beneficial effects from participating in the course lasted. Four years after taking the course, patients noted that pain levels were 19 percent lower and doctor visits had been reduced by 43 percent than before enrolling in the course.

3 Those who fail to benefit from arthritis self-management courses tend to be fatalistic people who believe that nothing can be done about their arthritis.

Measure Your Take-Charge Quotient

The developers of Stanford's Arthritis Self-Management Program created a test to help people assess their confidence in handling the consequences of their condition—a concept we refer to as TQ (take-charge quotient). Assessing your TQ will provide you with a report card on your role as a manager of your arthritis.

Take a few minutes to answer the questions on the next three pages, which measure your TQ for pain, functioning, and "other symptoms," and then tally up your score. A low TQ score

did you know

Pain reduction from taking the arthritis self-help course approximates the decrease in pain achieved by nonsteroidal anti-inflammatory drugs—and was above and beyond the pain relief from medical or surgical treatments that patients were receiving.

(between 10 and 60) in one or more areas means you could gain much from adopting a take-charge attitude.

Pain TQ

On a scale of 10 (very uncertain) to 100 (very certain)...

1. How certain are you that you can significantly decrease your pain?
2. How certain are you that you can continue most of your daily activities?
3. How certain are you that you can keep arthritis pain from interfering with your sleep?
4. How certain are you that you can make a small to moderate reduction in your arthritis pain by using methods other than taking extra medication?
5. How certain are you that you can make a large reduction in your arthritis pain by using methods other than taking extra medication?

(Average your scores for questions 1 through 5 to find your Pain TQ)

Functioning TQ

On a scale of 10 (very uncertain) to 100 (very certain), how sure are you as of now that you can...

1. Walk 100 feet on flat ground in 20 seconds?
2. Walk 10 steps downstairs in seven seconds?
3. Get out of an armless chair quickly, without using your hands for support?
4. Button and unbotton three medium-size buttons in a row in 12 seconds?
5. Cut two bite-size pieces of meat with a knife and fork in eight seconds?
6. Turn an outdoor faucet all the way on and all the way off?
7. Scratch your upper back with both your right and left hands?
8. Get in and out of the passenger side of a car without assistance from another person and without physical aids?
9. Put on a long-sleeve front-opening shirt or blouse (without buttoning) in eight seconds?

(Average your scores for questions 1 through 9 to calculate your Functioning TQ)

Arthritis Profile

William Ernest Henley

Few people better illustrate triumphing over adversity than William Ernest Henley. He was born in Gloucester, England, in 1849. At age 12 he was diagnosed with tubercular arthritis, a crippling and painful condition, and at age 16 doctors amputated his left leg below the knee.

Henley went on to finish his schooling and became a successful journalist in London. But at age 24, threatened with the loss of his other leg to tuberculosis, Henley went to Edinburgh and put himself under the care of the physician Joseph Lister, who saved Henley's leg.

During his long hospital stay, Henley wrote *Invictus*. The poem's theme of self-reliance in the face of overwhelming odds has inspired many people.

Invictus

Out of the night that covers me
Black as the Pit from pole to pole,
I thank whatever gods may be
For my unconquerable soul.

In the fell clutch of circumstance
I have not winced nor cried aloud
Under the bludgeonings of chance
My head is bloody, but unbowed.

Beyond this place of wrath and tears
Looms but the Horror of the shade,
And yet the menace of the years
Finds, and shall find, me unafraid.

It matters not how strait the gate,
How charged with punishments the scroll,
I am the master of my fate:
I am the captain of my soul.

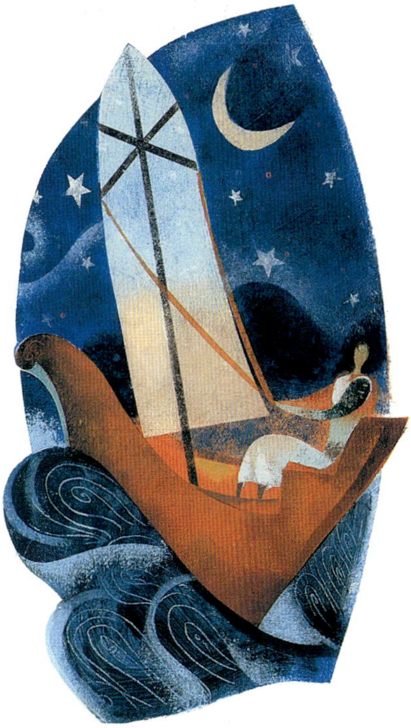

"Other Symptoms" TQ

On a scale of 10 (very uncertain) to 100 (very certain)...

1. How certain are you that you can control your fatigue?
2. How certain are you that you can regulate your activity so as to be active without aggravating your arthritis?
3. How certain are you that you can do something to help yourself feel better if you are feeling blue?
4. As compared with other people with arthritis like yours, how certain are you that you can manage arthritis pain during your daily activities?
5. How certain are you that you can manage your arthritis symptoms so that you can do the things you enjoy doing?
6. How certain are you that you can deal with the frustration of arthritis?

(Average your scores for questions 1 through 6 to calculate your "Other Symptoms" TQ)

what the studies show

Among more than 1,000 women, age 65 and over who were participating in Women's Health and Aging Study in Baltimore, Maryland, 115 reported that a doctor had diagnosed them with rheumatoid arthritis. But doctors at the Johns Hopkins Geriatric Center in Baltimore could verify the diagnosis in only 21 percent of these women. In describing their findings in the June 2000 issue of *The Journal of Rheumatology,* the doctors noted that women taking arthritis medication were especially likely to believe—mistakenly—that they had rheumatoid arthritis. The doctors also found that seven women who failed to report having rheumatoid arthritis did, in fact, have the disease.

What Does Taking Charge Mean?

Having a chronic disease like arthritis means that a cure probably isn't possible. In all likelihood, you will have arthritis for the rest of your life, so you will have to manage the problem one way or another—the choice is up to you.

One unfortunate but all-too-common reaction to a chronic disease is simply resigning oneself to it, a condition psychologists refer to as learned helplessness. A somewhat better management style is merely doing whatever your doctor tells you to do. The best approach of all—the one most likely to ease your pain, improve your mobility, and allow you to live life to the fullest—is to manage your arthritis in a positive way: in short, to take charge of it.

The CEO of your health. Taking charge of your arthritis is not that much different from being a manager in the business world. For example, top managers rely on consultants when making a decision. In your case, those consultants include family members and friends and, of course, health-care professionals including your physician, pharmacist, or physical

The ABC's of Self-Empowerment

Those who have taken charge of their arthritis live by several guiding principles:

- The patient's experience with his disease is unique—different from anyone else's who has ever had the disease—and so no single treatment will work for everyone.
- The patient, not his doctors, is the true expert when it comes to assessing how the disease is affecting him and how well treatments are working.
- The patient, who must live with his disease every day, is the person best qualified to take charge of his treatment.

therapist. But ultimately, all they can really offer you is advice. Since you are the manager of your arthritis, it's up to you to put their recommendations into action.

A caveat: Although arthritis self-help courses are often useful, they're not for everyone, and you may not want to follow the eight-step program we describe. But even if you're not a program person, you may find that pursuing just a few of the steps—getting to know your problem, for example, or thinking about your long-term goals—can make an important difference in the way you feel.

Becoming a Skilled Patient

Because you are a take-charge person, you need to equip yourself with the tools that are proven to ease symptoms: exercises and drugs to reduce pain, assistive devices and surgical techniques for improving mobility, visualization techniques for improving your mood, and many others. But to get the most out of each of them, you need to become a skilled patient.

Once you have learned and mastered the following eight steps, you'll be well on your way to controlling your arthritis—now and in the future, as well as during the inevitable ups and downs you may confront as your symptoms wax and wane.

1 Get to know your problem

Studies show that the better an arthritis patient understands her disease, the more likely she is to overcome it. You may think

Getting Acquainted with Your Pain

A big part of getting to know your arthritis problem is gaining a better understanding of how pain affects your life. One way to do that is to keep a pain diary.

About three times a day, pause in your activities, "take inventory" of your pain, and write down your observations. On a scale of 0 (no pain) to 10 (the worst pain you've ever had), how bad is the pain right now? What is its character—throbbing, burning, aching, stabbing? How does the pain make you feel emotionally—frustrated, hopeless, angry? Also, jot down what you were doing when you stopped to fill in your diary, and what you did to relieve the pain.

you're already quite knowledgeable about your condition, especially if you have been living with it for an extended period. After all, having lived with something for many years—whether it's a son, daughter, or disease—might lead you to assume that you're intimately familiar with it.

But what you think you know about your arthritis—what has caused it, how to treat it or prevent it from worsening—may not be true, or may be based on outdated information. In fact, you may not even have the disease you think you have. Even if your symptoms resemble those of your relative's or neighbor's, you may have an entirely different type of arthritis—or even a health problem that isn't arthritis.

Get a proper diagnosis. Receiving a diagnosis of arthritis certainly is not welcome news. But at least you now know the cause of your pain, stiffness, or disability. Armed with that knowledge, you can take the first steps toward overcoming the disease and its symptoms.

So, if you haven't already done so, your first step in taking charge of your condition should be to get a definitive diagnosis of your problem. If you are unsure about what type of arthritis you have—or whether you even have it—make an appointment with a doctor, who can evaluate you. Chapter 4 (*Working with Your Doctor*) tells you about the physicians who are qualified to diagnose arthritis.

Once you're sure about what type of arthritis you have, Chapter

2 (*Know Your Arthritis*) can help you become an expert on it. The chapter takes you inside the joints where problems arise and offers comprehensive descriptions of the major arthritic conditions: osteoarthritis, rheumatoid arthritis, and fibromyalgia, as well as less common but important ailments like gout and lupus. You will also read the latest findings on causes, diagnostic techniques, and treatments.

One Patient's Learning Curve

Consider the case of Jim, a 60-year-old grandfather. Recently, Jim realized that the "twinge" he had first noticed in his left knee a few years ago had by now become much worse. The knee was stiff for a good 15 or 20 minutes after he got out of bed in the morning. Walking for more than a block or so caused sharp, intermittent pain. Jim had always prided himself on being physically active, yet now his painful knee was preventing him from doing the things he loved—from playing catch with his grandson to going bird-watching with his wife.

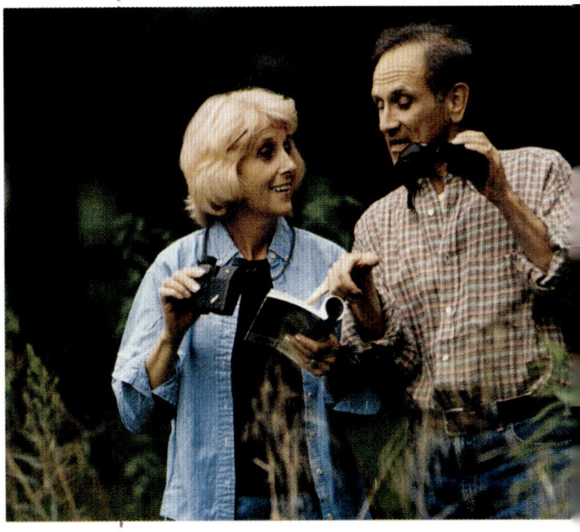

Jim regretted having to withdraw from the activities that had brought him joy. But he figured that aches, pains, and stiffness were a normal part of getting older—something he would just have to live with.

What the doctor discovered. Jim's wife, however, had noticed that her husband was becoming increasingly depressed as his knee problems worsened. She urged him to find out whether anything could be done. So Jim made an appointment with a rheumatologist, a doctor who specializes in treating arthritis and related conditions that affect the joints.

After taking Jim's history and doing a physical exam, the doctor told him that he had osteoarthritis of the knee. But he tempered the diagnosis with some good news: Many treatment options were available—not only for preventing the pain and stiffness in his knee from worsening but also for reducing those symptoms and giving Jim back his active life.

Jim made a second appointment with the rheumatologist to discuss his condition and his possible treatment options in more detail. In the meantime, he began reading this book to learn more about the causes of osteoarthritis and the take-charge approach for gaining control of it.

2 Choose your long-term goal

People with arthritis have a wide range of goals, from the unrealistic ("I want to be cured") to the vague ("I want to feel better") to the specific and realistic ("I want to climb the stairs unaided"). Specific, realistic goals are best.

In fact, you will learn that the take-charge approach to arthritis is based on setting and attaining specific goals. For one thing, you can readily tell whether or not you have attained a specific goal. You'll also find it's easier to motivate yourself to reach a specific goal than one that is vague or perhaps even undefinable.

Spend a few minutes thinking about your goals, and write them down on the lines on the opposite page. Try to list your goals in their order of importance to you, and try to choose goals

How to Be Goal-Oriented

Margaret A. Caudill, M.D., Ph.D., a leading pain specialist at Harvard University and New England Deaconess Hospital in Boston, says that every self-management goal should be:

Measurable. Define it in numerical terms if possible. Wrong: I'll develop better sleeping habits. Right: I will go to bed by 10 on most nights.

Realistic. Can you meet it, even if you are having pain? Wrong: I will catch up on my work without getting tired and hurting. Right: I will stretch and do hand-relaxing exercises for five minutes every hour.

Behavioral. It should be a specific action that you can take. Wrong: I will be more upbeat. Right: Whenever I feel hopeless, I will do a relaxation exercise and redirect my thoughts.

"I"-centered. Make it something you—not your mate, your children, or your employer—will do. Wrong: Everyone will give me time for my shower. Right: I will take a hot shower every morning.

Desirable. Is the effort worth the reward? There is no right or wrong here; just pay attention to yourself.

GOALS

1 ______________________

2 ______________________

3 ______________________

4 ______________________

that are measurable. Your most important goal is the one you should work toward first.

Before Jim's next appointment with his rheumatologist, he sat down to write out his goals. He tried to think of changes that would be especially valuable in transforming his life. He soon realized that one goal—walking a relatively long distance without knee pain—held the key to achieving several other goals. It also had the virtue of being measurable and realistic. So he listed this as his number-one goal, along with several others:

1 *Be able to walk a mile without knee pain*

2 *Go bird-watching with my wife, Sharon*

3 *Play catch with my grandson, Sean*

4 *Work in the garden again*

3 Decide on a strategy

Now that you have chosen your goals, it's time to formulate your arthritis strategy—the treatment approaches for achieving those goals.

Learning to pick and choose. In devising their strategy, arthritis patients obviously have many approaches to choose from. Arthritis often responds to some form of drug treatment. Alternative approaches, such as dietary supplements or perhaps mind-body treatments, also do the trick for some patients. Exercise helps most types of arthritis; surgery is an option when disability is severe.

As the manager of your arthritis, you should select the approaches that have the best chance of being successful for you. You may want a strategy that combines several different approaches, all of which may help you attain your long-term goal. Even if one approach is only modestly successful, others may prove more effective.

Think Strategically

With your goals in mind, think about the treatment approaches that might help you attain them. Reading the later chapters in this book can help you choose the approaches best suited to you and your condition.

As CEO of your arthritis, feel free to make use of consultants as you narrow down your list of treatment options to one or more that have the best chance of resulting in success. Your doctor, family members, and friends may all have opinions on approaches that are most likely to work for you. Just remember that you are the one who should have the final say on the treatments you use.

Treatments you'll stick with. Try to choose treatment approaches that you'll have a good chance of sticking with. So if you've always hated exercise, don't include it as one of your treatment approaches. But you may be enthusiastic about a cognitive approach that includes relaxation, guided imagery, or other mind-body techniques.

Once you've decided on some possible approaches, write them on the lines below. Try to list them in the order in which you'd be most likely to use them.

APPROACHES

1 ______________________

2 ______________________

3 ______________________

4 ______________________

Jim Chooses His Strategy

Jim learned about a number of possible approaches for treating osteoarthritis of the knee. He wrote down four that particularly appealed to him and shared them with his rheumatologist at his next appointment:

1. *Take pain-relieving drugs*
2. *Lose 10 pounds*
3. *Strengthen quadriceps muscles*
4. *Get hyaluronic-acid injections in his knee*

Now it was time to strategize: What treatment approaches would be best for reaching his goal of walking a mile without pain? Together, Jim and his doctor reviewed the benefits and drawbacks of the potential approaches that Jim had selected.

Take pain-relieving drugs. Jim had learned that the recently introduced COX-2 pain relievers (Celebrex, Vioxx, or Mobic) pose less risk of stomach upset than standard NSAIDs such as ibuprofen—an important consideration for him. But because Jim had an active stomach ulcer, his doctor advised him against using any type of NSAID, including the COX-2's. So Jim eliminated drug treatment as a strategy.

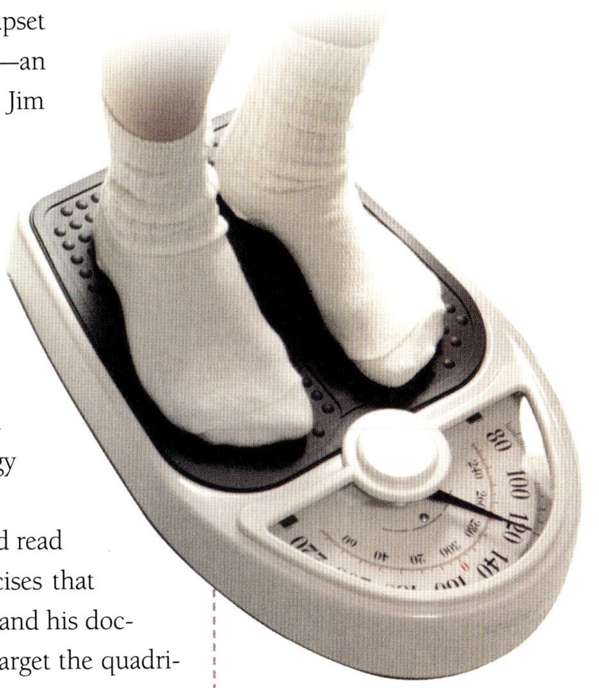

Lose 10 pounds. Jim had been overweight since he was a teenager. He knew that shedding excess pounds can do much to alleviate knee pain. His doctor agreed with Jim that losing 10 pounds could be a useful strategy for him.

Strengthen quadriceps muscles. Jim had read that arthritic knee pain responds well to exercises that strengthen the quadriceps (thigh) muscles. Jim and his doctor reviewed several exercises that specifically target the quadriceps muscles. The doctor also recommended two other exercises for strengthening Jim's leg muscles: regular walking and pedaling a stationary bicycle. As bonuses, walking and pedaling would improve Jim's aerobic conditioning and help in his weight-loss efforts by burning calories.

Get hyaluronic-acid injections in the knee. Jim knew that these shots offered the potential of reduced knee pain. But Jim's doctor noted that some rheumatologists still weren't convinced about the usefulness of the shots—which, in any case, were expensive (typically costing $1,000 for three physician-administered injections). Jim decided against the shots.

In the end, Jim decided to focus on two treatment approaches for relief of his knee pain: lose 10 pounds and strengthen his quadriceps muscles. Now that he had defined his arthritis strategy, it was time to pursue his goal in a systematic way.

4 Draw up your weekly take-charge plan

Take-charge planning is a means of reaching your ultimate goal through a succession of short-term goals. Think of the plan as a weekly contract that you make with yourself. Each week you assign yourself a series of specific actions, then build on your accomplishments from week to week. Ideally, someone who could climb only five stairs at week one will be climbing three flights after several weeks.

Boning Up: Invest in a daily planner to help schedule all of your activities —and schedule in rest periods, too.

Buying into the contract. The contracting process may seem burdensome at first. But once you get into the habit, you will find that it is well worth the effort. Your weekly successes will help convince you that you can indeed take charge of your arthritis and overcome the restrictions that the disease has imposed on you.

In creating your weekly plan, you will draw upon the actions that are part of your treatment approach. So if you have decided on a weight-loss approach, your plan will include weight-loss actions: eliminating between-meal snacks, for example, or walking to burn up calories.

Success is in the details. The key to a successful plan is to make your actions very specific (so they will be easier to repeat) and measurable (so you can easily score your success in completing them). If "walking" is one of your actions, for example, you should specify when you intend to walk ("before breakfast"), where ("around the block"), how often ("Monday, Wednesday, and Friday"), for how long ("10 minutes").

If you make your plan too ambitious, you may become discouraged by failure. On the other hand, you won't make progress if your plan is too modest. Ideally, try to include actions that are achievable but that may require a little effort. Once you've fulfilled those actions, you can write in slightly more ambitious actions for next week's plan.

Jim Makes a Plan

Jim's weekly take-charge plan incorporated both of his treatment approaches—losing weight and exercising. Since Jim had been a confirmed couch potato, his doctor gave him some good advice: "Set modest short-term goals during the first week. Perform each action just a few times, for just a few minutes, or at a low intensity. You'll have ample opportunity to make things more strenuous in the coming weeks, as your body adjusts to exercise."

Together with his doctor, Jim settled on three actions he would take during his first week. He would do some more often than others. His take-charge plan for exercise looks like this:

did you know

Moving around a bit at least every two hours can fend off stiffness. If you sit too much, get out and take a walk. If you stand for a prolonged time, enjoy a few moments off your feet. Set an alarm clock to remind yourself to take breaks.

Plan

Day	Action	Where	Time	Results
Monday	• *Leg flexes* • *Stationary bike*	*Bedroom* *YMCA*	*Mornings before* *work—After work*	✓ ✓
Tuesday	• *Walk around the block*	*Sheridan Park*	*Lunchtime*	✓
Wednesday	• *Leg flexes* • *Stationary bike*	*Bedroom* *YMCA*	*Mornings before* *work—After work*	✓ –
Thursday	• *Walk around the block*	*Sheridan Park*	*Lunchtime*	✓
Friday	• *Leg flexes* • *Stationary bike*	*Bedroom* *YMCA*	*Mornings before* *work—After work*	– ✓
Saturday	–	–	–	
Sunday	–	–	–	

Your weekly take-charge form. In writing up your weekly take-charge plan, be as specific as possible. State what you plan to do, how much you intend to do, when and where you will do those actions, and how many days a week you'll do them.

Plan

Day	Action	Where	Time	Results
Monday				
Tuesday				
Wednesday				
Thursday				
Friday				
Saturday				
Sunday				

5 Put your take-charge plan into action

Now comes the hard part: following through on the weekly plan that you've devised. Be prepared to do some work, and perhaps even make some sacrifices.

Jim Springs into Action

Jim found that setting aside time to exercise several days a week wasn't easy. As for the challenges of his weight-loss approach, he had a very hard time giving up the premium ice cream he was accustomed to having after dinner every night.

BONING UP: **If you haven't exercised in awhile and are apprehensive about taking the plunge, consult an expert. A physiatrist (a physician who specializes in rehabilitative medicine) or a physical therapist can help you design an exercise program tailored to your physical condition and your goals.**

Jim found that taking charge of his arthritis meant first taking charge of himself—and readjusting the way he had been living. "Old habits die hard," the saying goes, and adopting new ones can be even harder. Jim discovered that embracing new habits took persistence, but was worth the effort.

How Jim changed. Jim had to wean himself off some of his favorite television shows in order to fit in his exercise sessions. But he didn't forgo the tube completely—he simply taped the shows on his VCR and watched them later. When it came to giving up his full-fat ice cream fix, he downshifted into lower-fat varieties for several months and then, as his tastebuds acclimated to the "thinner" taste, moved into fat-free brands.

Jim also learned to be patient. His arthritis didn't develop overnight, so he realized that he shouldn't expect rapid improvement, either. It took him time to master the necessary skills. And even after he put his take-charge plan into practice, it took several weeks before he started noticing improvements. But he eventually attained those goals that he wished for but that were previously out of reach.

"I hated contracting when I took the self-help course. But now, as a course leader, I see that contracting is what changes people the most. It helps them find for the first time that they have control over their arthritis and can do things they never expected."

—Sharon Dorough,
arthritis self-help course leader

Getting Started

How many actions should you pack into your weekly plan, how often should you do them, and how much effort should you expend on them? The best advice is to take things slow and easy.

How many actions? Schedule just one or two actions for your first week. Beginning with just a couple of actions increases the odds that you will follow through on your assignment and that your weekly take-charge plan will develop into a habit.

How often will you do them? Doing something every day can be tedious as well as tiring. Probably the optimal frequency for any action is three to four times a week. The one exception is medication, which may need to be taken every day.

BONING UP: Practice patience when it comes to determining if a drug is relieving pain. NSAIDs require a one-or two-week trial to see if they work; slower-acting drugs such as gold may require six months.

How much will you do? Take your present condition as your starting point and progress gradually from there. If your knees start to hurt after you walk one block, your first plan should not call for walking a mile. On the other hand, you don't want to be so conservative that you don't make progress. As with so much in life, moderation is the best policy.

6 Monitor your progress

As you follow your take-charge plan during the week, gauge whether you've met each day's goals. You can do that directly by checking off the actions you have completed. Closely following up in this way gives you rapid and helpful feedback.

You should congratulate yourself if you've conscientiously stuck with the plan. But don't be hard on yourself if you have scored some incompletes. Instead, write out the same take-charge plan for the following week and see if you can do better.

Making progress, inch by inch. You may not be able to detect progress day to day, but an effective plan should produce

did you know

Changing behavior is a process, not a one-shot deal. It takes most people about 10 weeks to make significant changes in the way they handle pain, for example, and another six months until they are past the point that they risk backsliding.

small improvements each week. How do you assess such progress? You need to step back a bit and regularly take stock of how you're doing. That way, you can assess whether your efforts are making a difference—that they are moving you steadily toward your goal. One way to do this is through the use of "progress points."

Progress Points: Useful Milestones

In carrying out the actions in your take-charge plan—"walk around the block for a half hour before dinner each night," for example—you achieve the short-term goals that you want to build on, week by week.

Unfortunately, meeting your short-term goals does not mean you are making progress from week to week. You may feel that you're moving forward when actually you're running in place. Using progress points can help overcome this problem. They allow you to tell whether your combined actions are working and you are "on course" with your weekly actions.

Jim takes stock. Jim's take-charge plan incorporates a weight-loss approach. According to experts, losing one pound a week is a reasonable weight-loss goal for overweight people. Now Jim has a progress point —"lose one pound this week"—that can help him decide how strenuous his weight-loss actions should be.

A person can lose one pound in a week by burning up 3,500 more calories than he or she takes in. So Jim's plan might consist of a low-fat menu and fat-burning exercises that, together, make a 3,500 calorie difference. Simply by weighing himself at the end of the week, Jim was able to monitor his progress and the success of his plan.

caution

Don't overexert yourself if your take-charge plan involves exercise. To keep exertion within safe limits, exercise at an intensity that allows you to speak without gasping for air.

7 Adjust your action plan

If at first you don't succeed…maybe it's time to redo your plan. Perhaps your short-term goals are too ambitious and you need to scale back or allot yourself more time for completing them. With progress points (discussed above), you can gauge whether your take-charge plan needs to be adjusted.

If your progress point called for losing one pound last week and you lost only half a pound, perhaps you need to intensify your actions. If you lost more than a pound, maybe you're working too hard and need to moderate your actions. Either way, your progress point has "told" you that you need to fine-tune your action plan.

Jim Makes Adjustments

Sometimes the best progress point is how you feel. Jim's plan called for doing two sets of leg flexes to help strengthen the muscles around his knee. At the end of the first week, his thigh muscles were very sore.

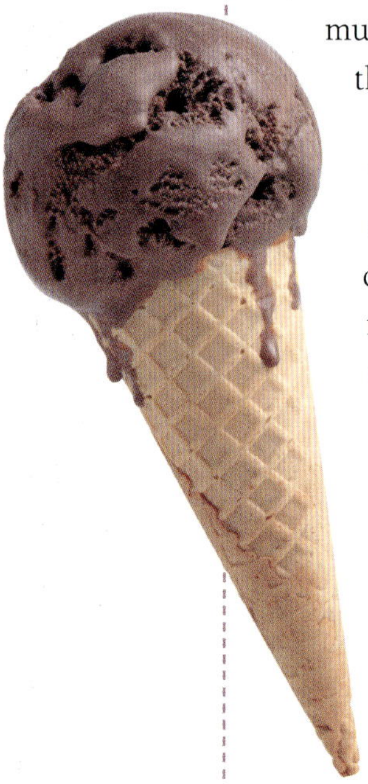

Jim's body was obviously sending him a message: "I'm not accustomed to this much exertion." So he decided to reduce his leg-flex regimen from two sets to one for the following two weeks. After that, if he experienced no muscle pain, Jim would try to resume doing two sets of leg flexes each day.

Jim also found that the transition from low-fat ice cream to fat-free was something he couldn't do easily. After a bowl of fat-free cherry vanilla, he still found himself loitering in the kitchen for an additional sweet treat to make up for his unsatisfying scoops of uncreamy ice cream.

So he explored the ice-cream section in his local supermarket and found that several premium ice cream companies made low-fat (three grams of fat) varieties that were indeed creamier tasting and more palate-pleasing than fat-free. He switched ice creams, and cut back on the number of scoops.

Correcting your course. These sorts of mid-course corrections not only help you move toward your goal but also sharpen your coping skills. People with arthritis constantly confront uncertainty: Flares and setbacks, unfortunately, are a "normal" part of the disease. A big part of taking charge of arthritis is becoming skilled at recognizing problems and working around them.

Boning Up: **If you have arthritis of the hands, stock up on pain relievers and vitamins without a child-protector cap. The caps can be hard to open for those suffering from such a condition.**

If you are a typist, for example, and morning stiffness in your fingers is interfering with your job, the best solution may be to modify your activities: arrange to start your workday later, for example, or build in frequent and regular breaks. Learning to adjust your plan as necessary can help you develop the flexibility needed to take charge of your arthritis.

8 Building on your success

In a way, building on success is the secret to gaining control over your arthritis. The take-charge approach hinges on achieving small successes week by week—until you arrive at an ultimate goal that may at first have seemed out of reach.

This time-tested formula helps explain why people who develop a successful plan for themselves tend to stick with it. The success you achieve one week has a beneficial effect not only on your joints but also on your attitude—helping you build confidence in your ability to manage your disease and overcome its limitations.

Little Victories

Build rewards into your plan, so that obtaining those rewards requires that you successfully complete an action. Jim, for example, loved to buy his daily newspaper on his lunch hour. So when he designed his daily lunch-hour walk, he made sure that it took him past a newsstand. For Jim, buying a newspaper was his way of rewarding himself for successfully completing that daily walk.

A final suggestion: Give yourself some time off for good behavior. Focusing on your arthritis every day may seem praiseworthy but can contribute to burnout. You'll have a much greater chance of reaching your goals if you give yourself a day or two off every week.

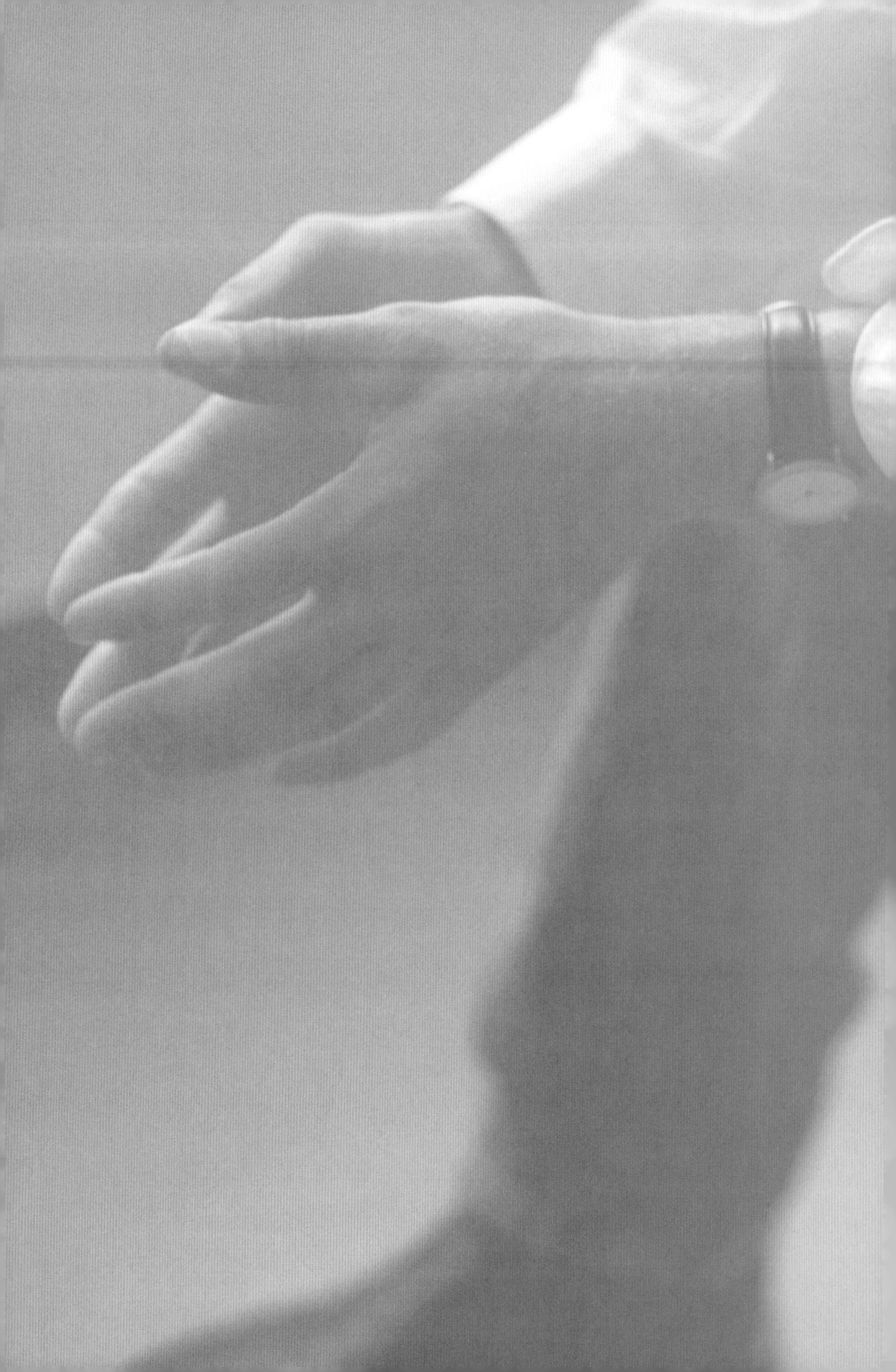

4 Working with Your Doctor

Many doctors today not only allow but even welcome their patients' input into treatment decisions. This is especially true for doctors who treat chronic diseases such as arthritis, for which there is no standard treatment or cure.

KEY CONCEPT

You are the manager of your arthritis. You enlist the experts—the physicians and other health-care members—listen to their treatment recommendations, and decide on the course of action.

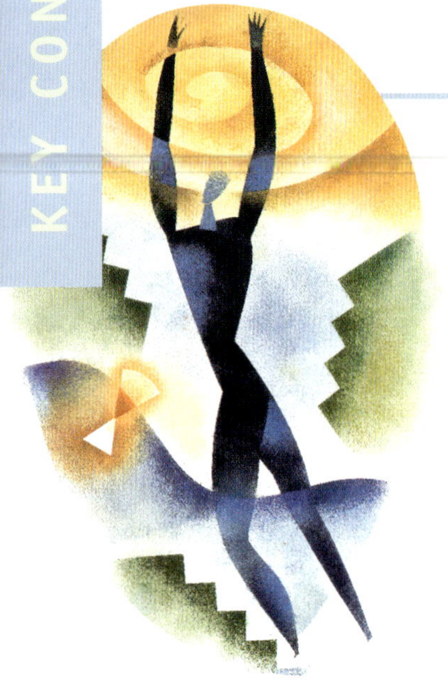

Doctor As Consultant

Although many doctors no longer consider themselves all-knowing authorities—a product of the new doctor-patient relationship that has evolved during the last several years—doctors' actions may still interfere with their intentions. Recent studies have found that conversations between doctor and patient more often resemble lectures than joint efforts to agree on a course of treatment.

Be assertive. Clearly, there is a need for patients to be more assertive in their dealings with doctors. For you, that means adopting a take-charge approach in your interactions with the physicians and other health-care professionals involved in your care. It encompasses:

- Deciding whether you could benefit from being under the care of a doctor in the first place
- Selecting a doctor whose expertise and personality meet your needs
- Participating in the diagnostic workup during your initial visit to the doctor's office
- Insuring you get the information you need from the limited time you may have during visits with your doctor
- Enlisting other health-care professionals in your effort to overcome your illness and improve your quality of life

As you assemble and work with the members of your health-care team, remember that you are the most important

Communicating with Your Doctor: Tips and Strategies

1 Make eye contact. Wait until you can make eye contact before you start talking about your problem. Doctors frequently enter the examining room reading your chart rather than addressing you.

2 Go from general statements to specific statements. Doctors have been taught to think this way.

3 Go from subjective (what you feel) to objective (information you can see, count, or touch). Your doctor's thought pattern is also moving in this way.

4 Always explain how your problems affect your life, work, relationships, sleep, etc. This will help elicit the doctor's compassion, help her realize she's treating a person, not just a disease.

5 Pause between parts of your story. This will allow your doctor to take notes and ask questions.

—From the book *Don't Let Your HMO Kill You*

person involved in your treatment. As someone who has taken charge of his or her arthritis, you are not "putting yourself under the care" of anyone. Instead, you are the manager of your arthritis and, the truth is, you will be the one carrying out the mutually agreed upon treatment decisions.

Do You Even Need a Doctor?

For people severely affected by arthritis, or diagnosed with a type of arthritis (such as rheumatoid arthritis) that must be carefully monitored, the answer to this question is clearly yes: They need a physician and the drugs that only physicians can prescribe to ease their symptoms and prevent the damage to their joints from worsening.

what the studies show

A study of medical visits found that doctors allow patients to talk for an average of only 18 seconds before interrupting them—and then spend less than two minutes of a 20-minute session sharing information with patients.

But for other people with arthritis—perhaps even the majority—whose symptoms are mild and manageable, the decision about whether to consult with a doctor isn't so obvious. For them, the take-charge approach advocated in this book—emphasizing self-care actions such as weight loss and exercise—may provide all the benefits they've been seeking. Or perhaps they did see a doctor years ago and have successfully followed through on the advice they received.

Doctor to the rescue. Some patients who have decided against seeing a doctor could genuinely benefit from it. Sometimes their opposition stems from ignorance of their

Facing the Fears of Arthritis

Some arthritis patients let fear rule their lives—as well as the management of their condition—when confronting it would help them progress to the next step of treatment or even to build a supportive health-care team. Here are three common fears along with strategies to put them into perspective:

Fear of the unknown. It is up to you, as we've already said, to educate yourself about your condition, ask questions of your doctor, and move into the daylight of enlightenment about your particular type of arthritis.

Fear of medications. It's a fact that all medications can cause side effects. Once again, knowing which medication works best for you, with a minimum of side effects, is the best defense against this fear. Every person responds differently to the same drug. Ask your doctor or pharmacist about the drug—and read up on your own—so you are comfortable with the medication choice you and your doctor have made.

Fear of depending on others. On one hand, you should actively pursue good nutrition, physical therapy, and other alternatives to help maintain your independence. On the other hand, your friends and family should be part of your health-care team. Your family will understand your suffering as no one else will. Share your thoughts and fears with family and friends, and they can help you work toward solutions.

disease or of treatments that are available. But all too often, such patients have a defeatist attitude toward their condition. They believe that it will inevitably worsen and so they must simply endure the accompanying pain and disability.

Since arthritis is rarely fatal, this misplaced stoicism usually isn't life-threatening. But by missing out on effective treatments, people may be subjecting themselves to needless pain and suffering. In addition, this neglect of their condition may allow joint damage to progress to the point that it can no longer be reversed except by surgery.

When to see a doc. The answer certainly is "yes" if you are experiencing one or more of the following symptoms:

- Persistent pain or stiffness after getting out of bed in the morning
- Soreness and swelling in any joint or in a symmetrical (both sides of the body) pair of joints
- Recurrence of the above symptoms, especially when more than one joint is involved
- Recurrent or persistent pain and stiffness in the neck, lower back, knees, and other joints
- Loss of weight, fatigue, and fever accompanied by joint pain

In addition, there are other, more general reasons to consider seeing a doctor:

- If problems with your joints are interfering with your daily life and your normal activities
- If you find yourself avoiding activities that you've previously loved doing
- If your joint pain is interfering with sleep
- If you find you are avoiding shopping or other social activities because you don't want to "slow everybody else down"
- If your joint pain or the limitations on your physical activity are making you feel anxious, helpless, or depressed

did you know

Muscle pulls, bone bruises, and ligament and other injuries can mimic the pain of osteoarthritis.

In the spirit of taking charge of your arthritis, it may be time to make an appointment with a doctor. Remember, you are under no obligation to agree with his or her recommendations. But you may find that working with a doctor is the crucial missing ingredient for making your take-charge program a success.

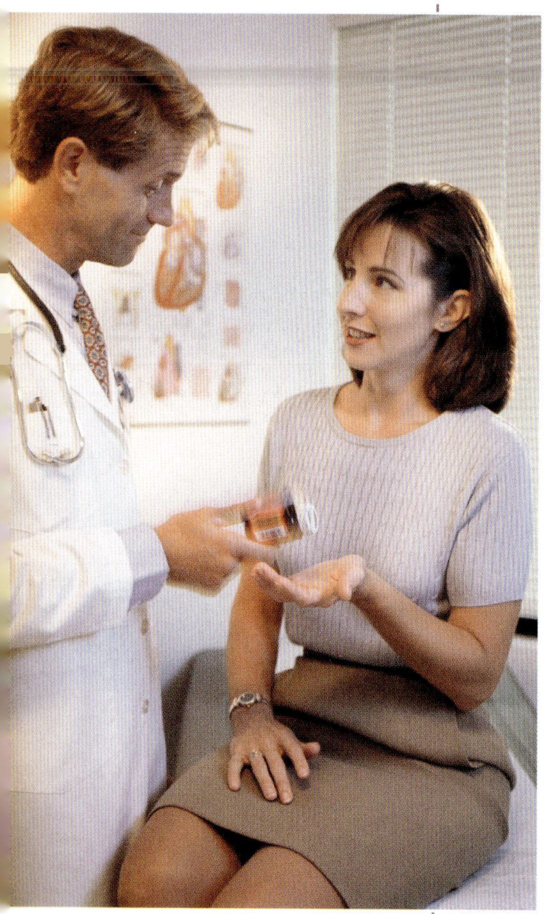

The Medical Marriage: How to Tie the Knot

For many common medical problems—colds, allergies, earaches, cuts and scrapes—our contact with doctors is episodic and usually brief: perhaps an initial appointment and a follow-up visit. Arthritis, on the other hand, is a chronic health problem, which means that a different treatment approach is needed.

Patients with arthritis may need regular and sometimes frequent visits over a period of years—to monitor the patient's overall physical and emotional health, to check for possible side effects from potent prescription drugs, and to deal with flares as they arise. Perhaps most crucially, there is no one "correct treatment" for a chronic disease like arthritis. As a result, managing a patient's disease may involve trying first one therapy, then another, or perhaps using several therapies in combination.

BONING UP: The patient's words are key when talking with a doctor. Studies of how doctors diagnose have shown that between 60 and 70 percent of all the information they need comes from the patient's medical history—an explanation of the medical problem in the patient's own words.

Symptom Sorting

Talking to your doctor about symptoms can be an art form when it comes to arthritis. Saying your knee hurts won't shed much light on your problem. Whenever possible, be specific.

For instance:

- how long the joint has felt painful or stiff
- what the pain is like—for example, constant or intermittent, or burning, throbbing, aching, or stabbing
- how the pain or stiffness has evolved—for example, mild at first and then increasingly severe, or severe from the very beginning
- what time of day the pain or stiffness is worse
- what makes the pain or stiffness in the joint better or worse
- how long the joint feels stiff after you get up in the morning
- whether the joint symptoms were preceded by illness or seemed to occur spontaneously
- how the symptoms are affecting your life—for example, do they prevent you from performing recreational activities that you've been able to do in the past, and do you feel frustrated or depressed because of this limitation?

List any other symptoms you've been experiencing, even if you don't think they could possibly be related to your condition. These would include fatigue, fever, chills, depression, or anxiety.

Are you compatible? As you can see, caring for someone with arthritis lends itself to a long-term partnership between patient and doctor. Indeed, you may end up becoming more familiar with your physician and his or her office than you would prefer!

As is true for marriage or for any other extended relationship, you should feel compatible with the physician you team up with. Whether you do feel comfortable depends a lot on the physician's personality—and your own.

Some patients thrive on the breezy, light-hearted approach, while others prefer that their doctors be sober, reflective, and unsmiling. But there is one "physician quality" that is crucially important to any arthritis patient—the ability to communicate. Few things are more important than a doctor's ability to explain things clearly. But as we'll see, communication is a two-way street—and you, as the patient, need to hold up your end of the relationship.

Know Your Physician

When it comes to choosing a physician for your arthritis, you basically have three choices: family physicians, internists, or rheumatologists.

Family physicians. Following medical school, FP's take post-graduate training in internal medicine, pediatrics, gynecology, orthopedics, and other fields. As their name implies, FP's learn about health problems that affect all family members of any age.

BONING UP: Don't always expect reassurance from your doctor. She won't say, "It's going to be okay" or "I'm sure it's nothing" until she is sure. She wouldn't want to reassure you only to have to break bad news later.

Second Opinions: Switching to a Specialist

The majority of arthritis patients have osteoarthritis. And fortunately, most cases of osteoarthritis are mild enough and uncomplicated enough that a primary-care physician—internist or family physician—can provide adequate care. But if your primary-care physician has treated you for more than a year, using a variety of different treatments, and your condition has still not improved significantly, then it's probably time to see a rheumatologist.

A good primary-care physician should respect your desire for a second opinion and should be willing to suggest a rheumatologist for you to see. If not, it may be time to get a different primary-care physician.

Diagnosed with Osteoarthritis? Ask These Questions

- What made you conclude that I have osteoarthritis?
- Can my symptoms have been caused by other diseases or conditions?
- If I do have osteoarthritis, is it primary or secondary?
- If it is secondary osteoarthritis, what other types of treatments could help eliminate the cause of the problem?
- Is there any joint deformity? If so, please tell me where and to what degree.
- Are there any bone spurs? If so, where?
- Have I lost range of motion in any of my joints? If so, where?
- Which treatment do you recommend? Why?

Internists. After medical school, internists take another three years of postgraduate training, which emphasizes treating serious health problems affecting adults. These include disorders of the heart, lungs, gastrointestinal tract, and the endocrine glands—as well as chronic diseases like arthritis.

Rheumatologists. These are physicians who specialize in diagnosing and treating arthritis of all types. Rheumatologists are internists who have taken two additional years of training in the treatment of arthritis and other problems affecting the joints.

The Match Game

Anyone with any form of inflammatory arthritis, including rheumatoid arthritis, should enlist a rheumatologist. Rheumatoid arthritis can be a very serious disease and is sometimes even life-threatening. It requires the expertise that only rheumatologists can provide. They are not only knowledgeable about the potent drugs used for treating rheumatoid arthritis but are also experts on their sometimes serious side effects.

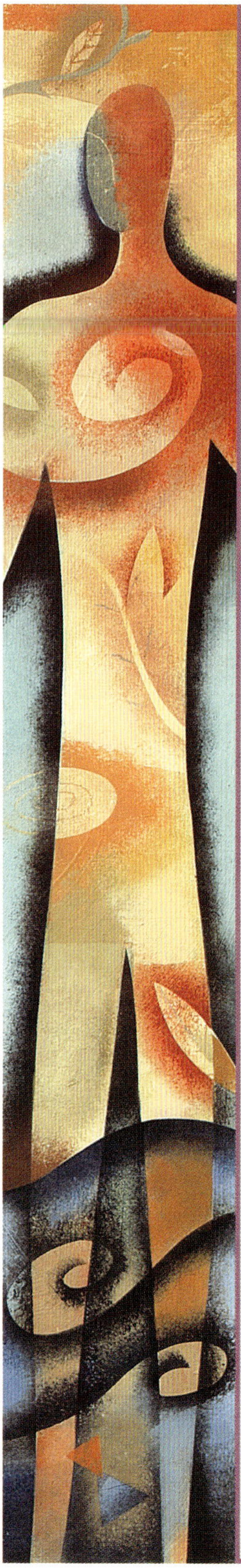

REAL-LIFE MEDICINE

New Knees: No Pain, More Gain

Forester Dan Gelbert has just spent a typical work day, hiking 10 miles through the North Carolina woods to carry out controlled burns of undergrowth. That's impressive enough for a 60-year-old—but truly amazing for someone with two artificial knees.

Some 40 years earlier, Dan had attended Duke University on a football scholarship. Twice in his football career he tore ligaments in his left knee and needed surgery to repair the damage. The torn ligaments led to cartilage damage—an all-too-common occurrence in athletes. In addition, the problems with his left knee caused Dan to favor his right leg, and the extra stress eroded cartilage there as well.

Soon Dan developed painful osteoarthritis in his left and right knees. Beginning about 10 years after college, the pain caused him to undergo six more operations on both knees—so-called debridements in which rough areas of cartilage are smoothed away.

Despite the pain, Dan was able to keep up his forestry work, which required him to be out in the field almost every day. He also continued sailing the 36-foot sailboat that he and his wife owned. But ultimately, the constant pain took its toll.

"Pain can begin to wear on you, but you don't realize that's happening after enduring it for so many years," says Dan. "It gets a little worse every day and creates problems, including psychological ones. For example, I didn't think I was depressed, but my wife and daughter were convinced I was. And that's understandable, because I hurt."

Dan realized he would need artificial knees if he wanted to maintain his strenuous forestry work and active lifestyle. And he wanted both knees operated on at the same time: "People who'd had the operation told me that if you only have one knee done, you'll never want to go through with the second procedure," he says.

Dan interviewed surgeons up and down the East Coast, but most would operate only on one knee at a time. That's because bilateral knee replacements, as they're called, greatly increase the risk of potentially fatal blood clots, perhaps because the operation takes longer or because most patients face a longer period of immobility when both knees are done together.

Finally, Dan persuaded an orthopedic surgeon in Virginia to operate on both of his knees. Dan's relative youth and good physical condition, the surgeon decided, would help speed recuperation and minimize risk. Dan received his two knee implants in June 1998—and indeed, he bounced back very quickly.

A key to Dan's successful outcome was working closely with his doctor. It was a partnership that began before Dan went in for surgery.

"A week before surgery, my surgeon requires that the patient and spouse come in to the office and spend over an hour getting educated," says Dan. "The doctor and his staff run through the complete operation with you. They also tell you where you're going to have your rehab work and how you should prepare your house for using a walker. What they showed us was exactly what happened. Working with the surgeon and following his recommendations to the letter was a big help for me in making a speedy recovery."

"I didn't think I was depressed, but my wife and daughter were convinced I was."

People normally remain hospitalized for four to six days after receiving a knee implant. But Dan—despite having two knees replaced—had recovered well enough to go home after three days. "Then I worked very hard at rehabilitation, which involves exercise and physical therapy that is very painful," says Dan. "But if you are going to walk again quickly, you have to do what they recommend."

Two years after Dan received his new knees, he pronounced himself "very pleased" with his condition. "Today I'm basically pain-free, and I feel that I've conquered my arthritis," says Dan. "If I had known that knee-replacement surgery was going to be so successful, I'd have done it 10 years ago."

Dan still faces a few limitations. "I can't climb fences easily, and I'm not supposed to bend my knees more than 90 degrees unless I have to," he notes.

Dan's advice for anyone planning to get knee implants: "Getting into good physical shape before going in for surgery can help you recover faster."

BONING UP: Osteoarthritis and other forms of arthritis are diagnosed after the pain has been present in a joint for a minimum of two consecutive weeks.

You should also be under the care of a rheumatologist—or at least get a consultation with one—if you have a complicated case of osteoarthritis that requires the use of several drugs. The rheumatologist may be able to devise a treatment regimen that makes you feel better than you've thought possible, with fewer side effects.

If your arthritis is mild or uncomplicated, a good initial choice for arthritis care may be a family physician or internist—perhaps the one you already have. He or she can usually diagnose arthritis based on your medical history, physical exam, X rays, and laboratory tests. As primary-care physicians, FP's and internists are trained to recognize when a patient's problems are beyond their realm of expertise and require the care of a specialist.

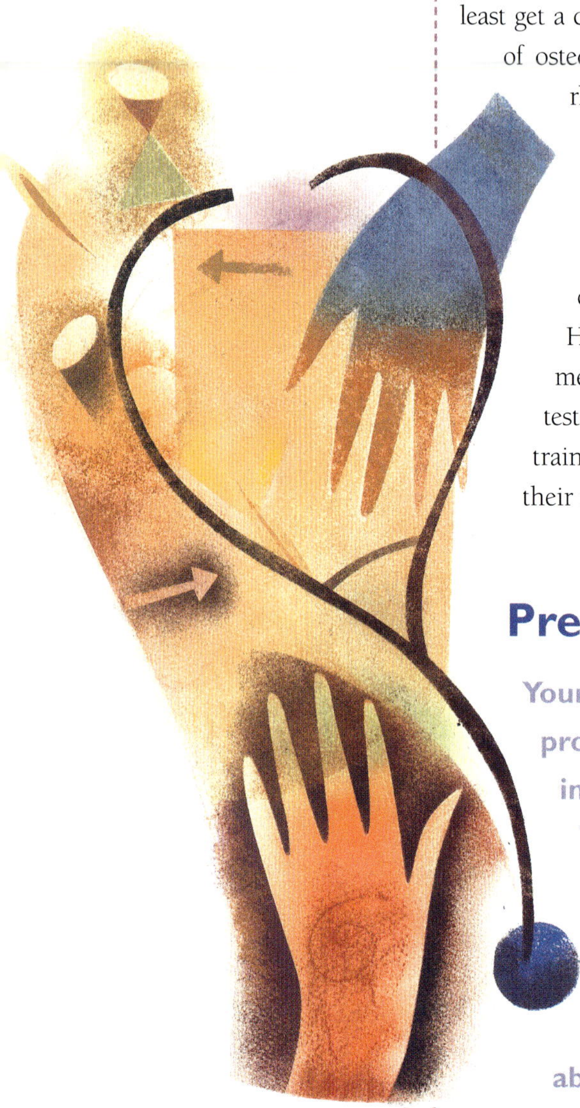

Preparing for an Initial Visit

Your first time in the doctor's office will provide your physician with basic but vital information about your physical condition. This meeting should help your doctor sketch out a medical portrait of you—in particular, whether you have arthritis and, if so, what type it is. But in addition, the first visit will allow you to learn a lot about your doctor.

During the visit, your doctor will ask you many questions about your health (i.e., take your medical history) and give you a physical exam. Based on findings from the history and physical, the doctor may take some X rays and collect blood from you for laboratory testing. Let's break this visit down into its components:

Your First Time: What You Should Take to the Doctor's Office

By arriving at your initial visit well prepared, you will help your doctor gain much better insights into your arthritis problems and how they can best be treated. A day or two before your appointment, compile several lists, each of them on a separate piece of paper:

A drug list. Your doctor will want to know what drugs you are now taking—not only for your arthritis pain but for any other health problems you may have. This list can give your doctor insights into your health and help prevent him from prescribing medications that might interact with other drugs you are taking. The list should include prescription drugs (your pharmacist may be able to give you a printout containing their generic and brand names), over-the-counter drugs such as antacids and pain relievers, and dietary supplements including vitamins, herbs, or any other "alternative" treatments that you are taking by mouth or rubbing on your skin.

A list of health problems. Since a medical history covers past and present health problems, your doctor will probably ask about health problems you have had previously. Make your list as complete as possible, even if it means including ailments you now regard as trivial. There is a good chance your doctor will also ask about health problems affecting your first-degree relatives (your parents, siblings, and children), so include this information as well.

A list of your symptoms. During the history, your doctor will ask you to describe your symptoms and then ask you specific questions about them. By jotting down this information ahead of time—when you don't feel as rushed as you might in the doctor's office—you will be able to give your doctor a fuller picture of the extent and severity of your arthritis.

The medical history. The patient history has traditionally been thought of as a one-way interrogation (although much friendlier than a police interrogation, and with no lawyers present), in which the doctor asks questions and the patient answers them. But ideally the history is a collaborative effort, and you should feel free to volunteer information that could give your doctor a better insight into your arthritis.

BONING UP: Get to the heart of your medical problem quickly. According to one study, patients who were allowed to talk uninterruptedly to their doctor about a problem spoke for $2\frac{1}{2}$ minutes—much too long considering that doctor's visits run, on average, 10 minutes these days.

The physical. After taking your history, the physician will then do a physical examination. In addition to performing the elements of a routine examination (taking your blood pressure and your pulse, listening to your heart), the physician will examine your joints to see how they function while you're sitting or standing still and when you walk, stretch, or bend.

Closely examining the affected joints, the physician will determine whether they are swollen and, if so, whether the swelling is due to thickened synovial (soft) tissue in the joint (which suggests rheumatoid or some other type of inflammatory arthritis) or instead is caused by bony swellings (bone spurs indicate that osteoarthritis is present).

Finally, a good diagnostician will look at the pattern of joint involvement: Pain or swelling in symmetrical joints (the joints connecting both big toes to the feet, for example) is often a tipoff for rheumatoid arthritis.

Laboratory tests. As we noted in Chapter 2, relatively few laboratory tests can actually help to diagnose the various types of arthritis. Instead, lab tests are useful mainly for ruling out other possible causes of joint pain, such as infections, side effects from drug treatment, or cancer.

did you know

- If your pain is worse after exercise, it may be due to joint alignment problems. If the pain tends to lessen after exercise, this suggests a need to improve muscle tone.
- Some diets—those high in red meats, for example—may worsen inflammatory types of arthritis. A vegetarian diet has been shown to help some patients with rheumatoid arthritis.

Physician-Patient: One Doc's View

"It's going to be a long relationship, and neither party should expect too much from the first encounter. A patient's questions should be answered as fully as time and reason allow, and the doctor should expect that the patient will be somewhat anxious.

"The patient shouldn't expect that the doctor can—or should try to—cover every aspect of the disease and all its possible outcomes during the first visit. The relationship is an evolving one, and much depends on developing mutual trust between doctor and patient.

"What the patient needs most during that first visit is an unhurried discussion of his or her symptoms, the diagnosis—if one can be made at that time—and the possible options for treatment."—John Hassall, M.D., professor emeritus of rheumatology, Royal Prince Alfred Medical Center, Sydney, Australia

X rays. These images can provide objective evidence that arthritis is present—and, if so, what type it is. For example, the x-ray images of joints affected by osteoarthritis and rheumatoid arthritis usually look quite different.

Getting the Most from Later Visits

Repeat visits to the doctor are a hallmark of all chronic diseases, including arthritis. As you undoubtedly know, most doctors have only a limited amount of time to spend with patients who come for routine visits. So you should make an effort to use that time wisely. Here are some practical tips for gaining maximum benefit from your visit.

what the studies show

When patients with chronic health problems—hypertension, diabetes, and peptic ulcers—were coached on how to become more assertive with their doctors, they reported better overall health and fewer limitations on their social life and work life due to illness.

Prepare some talking points

Just as you did before your initial visit, plan for your upcoming visit by thinking about the problems or questions that you have. Then write them down in the order of their urgency, so that you'll be sure that your most pressing issues will be dealt with. As a practical matter, don't include more than three questions or concerns on your agenda, since it's unlikely you'll have time to discuss more than that.

Remember why you are in the office

In a hit song from the 1960s, the singer announces that he "just dropped in to see what condition my condition was in." Before you decided to take charge of your arthritis, you may have approached your doctor visits that way—with you sitting passively as the doctor asked you questions, felt your joints, and told you whether you were doing well or poorly. How you felt was not something you thought was worth mentioning.

Office etiquette. Adopting a take-charge approach during doctor visits will help you get much more out of them. Telling your doctor how *you're* doing, how well the drug is working, whether the exercises are helping, and how you are feeling will benefit you and will make your doctor happier. And if you are having problems, you should volunteer that information and then spell out just what difficulties you are experiencing.

Women especially have trouble taking this assertive approach with physicians, for fear of offending or insulting them. But actually, most doctors much prefer that patients provide them with that kind of feedback. Only by working together in this way can patient and doctor develop the treatment approach that will be the best possible one for the patient.

> "Early on, I would go to the doctor just to see how I was doing....Now I know that my doctor was looking for me to tell him how I was doing, and not the other way around."
>
> —Sharon Dorough, arthritis patient

Clear up uncertainties

All too often, doctors talk in jargon when discussing issues with patients. Or they may simply fail to explain why they're recommending that you take a certain drug or stop taking another.

Whatever the reason, questions will almost inevitably arise during your visit—and what you don't understand could prevent you from gaining a better understanding of your arthritis. So don't be afraid to tell the doctor that you don't understand something or that you're confused. Most doctors won't mind going back over what they've said so that you can understand it.

Be a good reporter

When visiting the doctor, it's all too easy to make the forest-for-the-trees mistake: perhaps becoming so distracted by a technical term you didn't understand that you weren't tuned in when the doctor was discussing possible side effects from a new drug he was recommending.

Taking notes can help insure that important information doesn't get lost in the ether. Tape-recording the visit (with your doctor's permission) and then playing back the tape when you get home can also help. Or bring along a friend or family member for backup: Comparing notes with that person can help fill in details that you might have missed.

Building Your Team

It has become increasingly apparent that a patient's interests may best be served by a "treatment team." In this team approach, one doctor typically serves as physician-in-charge, coordinating the care administered by other physicians or health-care professionals. The team may include one or more of the following:

A nurse in a doctor's office or clinic can often provide information that the doctor missed, or clarify a comment the doctor made. A competent, caring nurse can answer questions about the side effects of a medication or get access to the doctor to provide an answer. Some nurses are trained in rheumatology and can help with modifications in the home, office, or even school to make your life a little easier. A nurse can become a counselor, friend, and an advocate for you.

Physical therapists prescribe exercises aimed at relieving pain and restoring lost muscle and joint function. In many cases, they can give you back the mobility you may have lost. They can work with you to create a personalized regimen consisting of stretching as well as strength and aerobic exercises.

did you know

All qualified occupational therapists should be registered with the American Occupational Therapy Association.

on the horizon

Several doctors in the United States have been experimenting with meniscus transplants. They theorize that restoring a damaged meniscus (the cushioning cartilage in the knee) with either donated tissue or synthetic materials may help to normalize the joint forces and prevent or slow osteoarthritis.

They sometimes recommend water therapy, relaxation techniques, even biofeedback. A course of physical therapy generally lasts just a few weeks, although long-term therapy may sometimes be recommended.

Occupational therapists evaluate patients' ability to perform work both inside and outside the home. With the occupational therapist's advice, you can learn new ways of doing old things—from housework to cooking a Thanksgiving meal. They often make suggestions for modifying the home and work environment so that you can function more efficiently and with less pain. Occupational therapists can also design and fit any splints or other devices you might need to support or protect weakened joints.

Nutritionists can also help you overcome the daily pains and aggravations of living with arthritis. When you are diagnosed with arthritis, how you eat and what you eat can significantly impact your pain and health. The nutritionist is there to explain the way foods interact, how the drugs you might be taking could deplete certain nutrients, and how vitamins might help. And, of course, proper nutrition will help you pare pounds—an essential task in reducing pain for many patients.

Orthopedic surgeons are physicians who perform surgery on joints, including arthroscopy and joint-replacement surgery. Primary-care physicians or rheumatologists may refer an arthrtis patient to an orthopedic surgeon if drugs fail to relieve pain or disability.

Physiatrists are physicians who specialize in rehabilitation medicine. Physiatrists can prescribe special exercise programs, crutches, or devices that protect the joints.

Psychiatrists, psychologists, and social workers can help arthritis patients cope with depression, anxiety, and other psychological problems that are often associated with having a chronic disease.

Family and friends are also vital resources in achieving your goals. Because arthritis is a long-term battle, you will occasionally need day-to-day help. When it is tough to get out of bed because your knees feel like hardened cement, a friend or family member can provide a gentle shove toward that hot bath or shower. When you boil it down, your family and friends have a vested interest in helping you take charge of your condition.

If you think you might benefit from a team approach, don't hesi-

When Surgery Is Recommended: Ask These Questions

- What surgery are you recommending?
- Please describe what happens during the surgery.
- Exactly how will I be better off as a result of this surgery?
- What is the normal range of outcomes from this type of surgery?
- Please describe all the side effects of this surgery.
- How long will I be in the hospital?
- How much pain will I experience, and what can be done to relieve it?
- Should I arrange to have someone help me when I return home?
- Will the surgery affect my ability to work?
- In what hospital will the surgery be performed? Is it noted for good surgical results?
- Do you have any books or pamphlets describing the surgery?
- Do you have any patients who underwent the same surgery that I can talk to?
- Can the surgery significantly affect or cure my osteoarthritis?
- Could the surgery make my condition worse than it is now?

tate to discuss the matter with your physician. Even better, suggest the specialist you have in mind—a physical therapist, for example—and ask if your doctor could recommend a particular individual.

Call for help. If your physician is unable to refer you to a physical therapist or other arthritis specialist, call your local chapter of the Arthritis Foundation and ask for their help. They have a directory of members belonging to the Arthritis Health Professionals Association. Too many cooks may spoil the broth, but having the right number of specialists working for you can help push you toward your goal of taking charge of your arthritis.

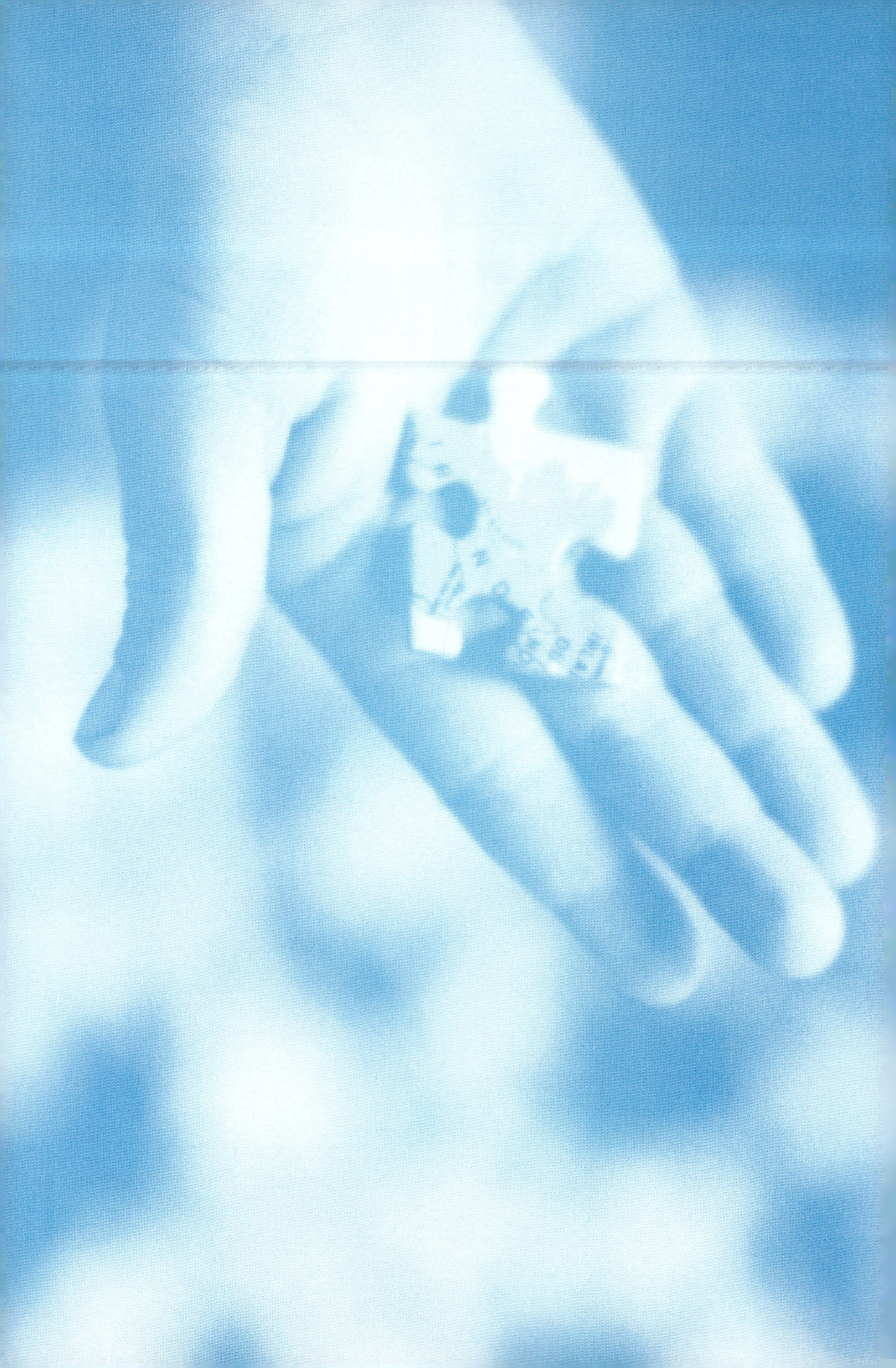

5 Treating Arthritis: Drugs and Surgery

There is an ever-increasing number of drugs that can combat the inflammation and pain of arthritis. There are also new surgical options when pain doesn't respond to medication. Choosing the right drug or surgical procedure can often mean the difference between living fully and being imprisoned by your condition.

KEY CONCEPT

Arthritis patients can choose from numerous drugs to relieve pain and stiffness. If one drug doesn't help or causes side effects, another is very likely waiting in the wings.

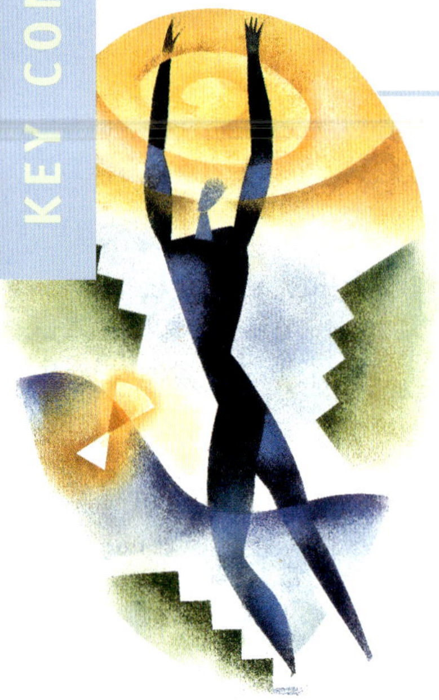

Mind Your Medications

All types of arthritis have two things in common: They affect the joints in some way, and they cause pain. So it's not surprising that many of the drugs used to treat arthritis help short-circuit pain.

Multiple options. They range from old reliable aspirin—used for more than a century—to several new and exciting drugs that have been available only since 1998. For the vast majority of arthritis patients who have osteoarthritis, the drug news is mixed. Although many medications can help relieve pain, no drug yet can do what OA patients need most: rebuild cartilage that has been damaged and lost over the years. (Certain dietary supplements may offer some help when it comes to restoring lost cartilage, as you'll see in Chapter 6.)

On the other hand, new drugs known as COX-2 inhibitors are much less likely to cause stomach irritation and bleeding than older arthritis drugs. Some of the newest and most promising medications are reserved for people with rheumatoid arthritis and other forms of inflammatory arthritis.

Take Your Medicine: Patient Education

One reason that so many medicines are manufactured for people with arthritis is that individuals respond differently to each one of them. There are currently some 30 brands of NSAIDs on the market, with about 20 more awaiting FDA approval. So chances are you will find a drug that will work for you. But no matter which medication you turn to, you should always bone up first: get the nuts-and-bolts information on safe dosages, side effects, and expense.

You and your doctor should weigh how much good a medicine can do for you against how bad its side effects may be. The prescribed dosage usually starts low, then increases to a level that either helps the arthritis or causes unpleasant side effects. If side effects do occur, the dosage can usually be reduced.

Taking charge of your arthritis requires that you take your medications properly, according to your physician's orders, and that you notify your doctor about any potential complications or side effects. And never let nagging pain seduce you into borrowing a medication from a friend who swears that it will work wonders for you. Interactions—some of them dangerous—can always occur.

did you know

Fewer than one person in 20 has to stop a medicine because of bad side effects; aspirin is an exception, with one in six taken off the drug.

Drug Etiquette: Taking Stock Before Taking a Drug

Beginning a new medicine: Ask about possible interactions with other drugs and if there are any special instructions relating to the absorption of the medicine: Is it important to take it between meals, with meals, or right at bedtime? Also, ask the doctor for the lowest dose of the drug that might still reduce your pain and inflammation. The lower the dose, the lower the chances of suffering serious side effects.

Side effects: Since many arthritis drugs can cause anemia, stomach ulcers, and other gastrointestinal side effects, as well as kidney and liver damage, make sure your doctor has you come into the office for lab tests. Also, don't mistake an allergic reaction for an adverse reaction: Allergic reactions usually result in hives or itching. Adverse reactions are often more serious.

Adding new medicines: When your doctor and you decide that a new medicine is needed, she should explain how the medicine is thought to work, what dose to take, the possible side effects, and the potential cost. In addition, your doctor should ask you to return in one to two weeks for a safety check. She should ask you about any side effects such as diarrhea, abdominal pain, headaches, blurred vision, or drowsiness.

BONING UP: When the physician or nurse asks you to come in for a safety check on a medicine, do it. A blood count, urinalysis, or a liver function test may be required, depending on the drug and its effect on you.

Acetaminophen: The First Choice for Pain Relief

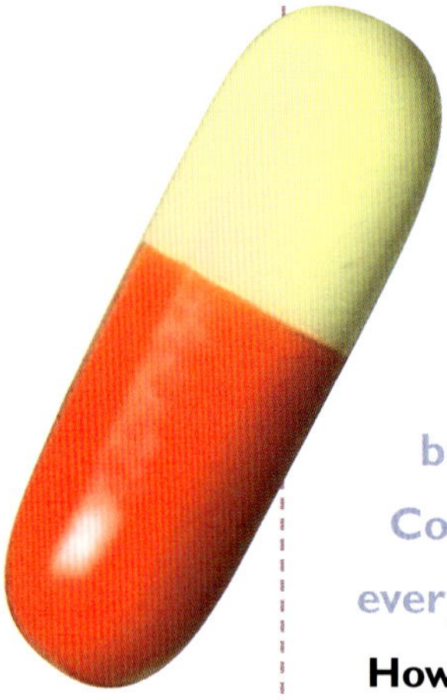

Sold under the brand names Tylenol and Panadol, among others, acetaminophen is effective for osteoarthritis patients who have mild-to-moderate joint pain. Acetaminophen has been available since 1955 and is now the nation's leading pain reliever. The medication is not only effective but is also among the safest drugs you can take. Considering the millions of doses consumed every year, it causes remarkably few side effects.

How it works. Acetaminophen relieves pain in a different way than nonsteroidal anti-inflammatory drugs, or NSAIDs. Aspirin, ibuprofen, and other NSAIDs block the body's production of prostaglandins, chemicals produced by the body that increase inflammation and pain. Acetaminophen, on the other hand, has no effect on prostaglandins; it works on the nervous system, raising the brain's threshold for pain.

The downside of acetaminophen is that it indeed has no effect on prostaglandins, and, as a result, will relieve only pain—not inflammation. So it won't be as effective as an NSAID against inflammatory types of arthritis. The upside is that by leaving all prostaglandins alone—including the "good" ones that protect the stomach lining—acetaminophen is much easier on the stomach than NSAIDs.

The Unsaids About NSAIDs

Until a few years ago, doctors routinely prescribed NSAIDs rather than acetaminophen for their arthritis patients. NSAIDs, however, can cause serious adverse effects, particularly gastrointestinal problems.

The inside scoop. Within a year of starting treatment with an NSAID, up to 4 percent of regular users develop stomach bleeding or painful ulcers. Prolonged use of NSAIDs also increases patients' risk for liver disease and kidney disease (problems that are more likely to occur in people over 70) and also for high blood pressure.

On top of the risks comes the expense: A month's supply of a prescription NSAID costs anywhere from $15 to $100; a month's supply of generic extra-strength acetaminophen, sold in 500-capsule bottles, costs about $5.

Gaining Respect

Recent research has shown that many arthritis patients don't need NSAIDs after all. Although inflammation is certainly the main cause of the pain and joint damage in rheumatoid arthritis, scientists now know that inflammation is only rarely present in osteoarthritis—by far the most common type of the disease. And when acetaminophen was matched up against powerful NSAIDs in clinical studies involving osteoarthritis patients, the over-the-counter pain reliever proved surprisingly effective.

Help for painful knees. One such study, published in *The New England Journal of Medicine* in 1991, involved 184 patients with chronic, persistent knee pain due to osteoarthritis. Acetaminophen was found to work as well as prescription-strength NSAIDs in relieving knee pain. This and other studies have shown that acetaminophen relieves mild-to-moderate osteoarthritis pain just as effectively as prescription NSAIDs—even in cases where the joints are actually inflamed.

Since acetaminophen worked as well as NSAIDs but without the serious risks of regular NSAID use, it made sense for osteoarthritis patients to try acetaminophen first. So in 1995, the American

did you know

Medicines sometimes stop working after months or years of providing pain relief. This is called tachyphylaxis. Although your doctor often can't tell you why this happens, he has just two options: increase the dose or prescribe a new medicine. In some cases, the failed medicine can be prescribed months or years later and be effective again.

Acetaminophen: More Virtues Than Vices

Compared with NSAID pain relievers, acetaminophen is:

- Gentler on the gastrointestinal tract and much less likely to cause stomach bleeding or ulcers
- Not a risk for raising blood pressure after prolonged use
- Less likely to cause liver or kidney disease after prolonged use
- Less likely to interact with other medications

College of Rheumatology changed its guidelines for the medical care of osteoarthritis and recommended that acetaminophen, at doses up to 4,000 mg per day, should be "the initial drug of choice" for treating osteoarthritis of the knee and hip.

did you know

In Europe, suppositories are a popular way of administering NSAIDs because they reduce stomach pain and nausea. They are less popular in the U.S. because Americans are uncomfortable about taking drugs rectally.

Next Drug, Please

Acetaminophen's gentleness on the gastrointestinal tract makes it the preferred first choice for easing the pain of osteoarthritis, which rarely involves inflammation (swelling, redness, and warmth). But if you have tried acetaminophen for a month and it fails to ease your pain, talk to your doctor about moving on to one of the NSAIDs.

Although NSAIDs do pose a greater risk for side effects, they may offer better pain relief than acetaminophen. You may also find that combining acetaminophen with an NSAID allows you to obtain pain relief with a lower (and safer) dose of NSAID than you would otherwise need. However, always talk with your doctor to find out if it is safe for you to combine two different pain relievers.

Precaution Primer

Despite its admirable safety record, acetaminophen can cause serious illness and even death. Regular users—those who take acetaminophen every day over many years—face an increased risk of liver or kidney damage. And both regular and casual users of acetaminophen can experience serious liver damage if they take high amounts of the drug while also consuming three or more alcoholic drinks a day.

BONING UP: Taking acetaminophen with food and avoiding alcohol can reduce your risk of kidney failure.

Watch the dosage. Problems with acetaminophen almost always result from doses far in excess of the maximum recommended dose of 4,000 mg per day. (But for older people and anyone with preexisting liver disease, even a modest overdose can be dangerous.)

One other caution: Be wary of acetaminophen if you are in the habit of fasting. A 1994 study in the *Journal of the American Medical Association* found that when people who have been fasting or who haven't been eating due to the flu or a stomach virus consume "moderate overdoses" of acetaminophen—between 4,000 mg (the maximum recommended dose) and 10,000 mg daily—they increase their risk for liver damage.

what the studies show

Most patients who take both acetaminophen and an NSAID for osteoarthritis say that the NSAID is more helpful against pain, according to a study in the April 2000 issue of *The Journal of Rheumatology*. On the other hand, acetaminophen was better tolerated: 33 percent of the patients continued taking acetaminophen for more than two years, versus only 21 percent for ibuprofen, 17 percent for naproxen, and 19 percent for diclofenac.

NSAIDs: Not Just Your Father's Aspirin Anymore

Nonsteroidal anti-inflammatory drugs, or NSAIDs, are effective for arthritis patients who suffer from pain and/or inflammation—particularly those with inflammatory types of arthritis such as rheumatoid arthritis and ankylosing spondylitis.

First-line drugs. If you are taking a drug for arthritis pain, you may well be taking one of the many NSAIDs that are now available. ("Nonsteroidal" means that these drugs do not include prednisone or other members of the corticosteroid family of drugs, which are also anti-inflammatory.) NSAIDs are used against arthritis pain and many other types of pain, including headache, menstrual pain, and dental pain.

caution

Patients with a history of asthma attacks, hives, or other allergic reactions to aspirin should avoid NSAIDs.

All the NSAIDs have one thing in common: They relieve pain in low doses, and pain and inflammation at high doses.

Taking NSAIDs— And Keeping Your Stomach Happy

Gastrointestinal irritation is by far the most common (and often the most serious) problem posed by NSAIDs. If you take an NSAID for your arthritis, you can do several things to make the experience more stomach-friendly:

1 Take the drug with a glass of water and during meals.

2 Don't lie down from 15 to 30 minutes after taking the drug.

3 Limit your alcohol intake to three drinks a day or less, since combining NSAIDs with heavy drinking increases the likelihood of gastrointestinal irritation.

4 Ask your doctor about instituting a drug holiday. Taking NSAIDs a few days on and a few days off can give the stomach some time to heal itself. If the pain and inflammation become too intense, acetaminophen may be an alternative during the off days.

5 Consult your doctor before mixing NSAIDs, even if both drugs are taken in low doses. Combining NSAIDs—especially in anti-inflammatory doses—can greatly increase the risk of stomach irritation.

6 If you take occasional doses of aspirin, products that contain antacids—"buffered" aspirin brands such as Ascriptin and Bufferin—may reduce stomach irritation, although they may not be gentler to the stomach with long-term use. Enteric-coated aspirin (Ecotrin) may also help, by preventing aspirin from dissolving in the stomach. It dissolves, instead, in the small intestine. On the other hand, the coating also means you'll have to wait longer for pain relief.

Many people with osteoarthritis take NSAIDs for pain relief—but most of them don't need high doses, since inflammation usually isn't present in OA. But for people with OA who also suffer with inflammation or who have any type of inflammatory arthritis, taking a high-dose NSAID to reduce inflammation can be extremely helpful, since the inflammation damages the joint and causes much of the pain.

The NSAIDs include over-the-counter medications that you are probably familiar with, such as Advil, Nuprin, Aleve, and Orudis KT. They also include higher-dose prescription versions of these drugs as well as many other prescription drug brands, such as Feldene, Relafen, and Clinoril. Old standby aspirin, which was first marketed in the U.S. in 1899, is also classified as an NSAID.

what the studies show

From 40 to 60 percent of people who chronically use either prescription or nonprescription NSAIDs develop shallow injuries ("erosions") in the lining of their stomach or small intestine. Between 10 and 30 percent of chronic users will end up with deeper injuries (ulcers).

The Pluses and Minuses of NSAIDs

NSAIDs work by preventing the body from producing pain-inducing chemicals called prostaglandins. They shut off the "bad" prostaglandins by blocking an enzyme called cyclooxygenase (COX) 2.

Double-edged swords. But unfortunately, in addition to blocking COX-2, standard NSAIDs also block the COX-1 enzyme, which produces "good" prostaglandins that protect the lining of the stomach and other parts of the gastrointestinal tract by regenerating their mucus lining. Without this mucus lining, the gastrointestinal tract can be damaged by acidic and caustic digestive fluids that are always present. Not surprisingly, NSAIDs in prescription-strength doses are more likely than nonprescription NSAIDs to cause problems.

BONING UP: **If you are at high risk for gastrointestinal complications, perhaps you should try diclofenac sodium (Arthrotec). It combines the NSAID diclofenac with misoprostol, man-made prostaglandins that help protect the GI tract.**

So while NSAIDs help relieve pain and inflammation, they can also cause major gastrointestinal problems, including ulcers and significant bleeding. In fact, every year in the U.S., NSAIDs kill at least 16,500 arthritis patients, send more than 100,000 patients to

caution

The American College of Rheumatology recommends that osteoarthritis patients should avoid indomethacin (Indocin), since some studies suggest that prolonged use of this powerful NSAID may hasten cartilage degeneration. It is not yet clear whether other NSAIDs can also damage cartilage.

the hospital, and cause gastrointestinal discomfort in many others.

But these statistics should be kept in perspective: NSAIDs are one of the most popular classes of drugs, and prescription NSAIDs alone are consumed by some 33 million Americans each year. Clearly, the vast majority of people who use NSAIDs don't experience serious complications from them.

Choosing the Right NSAID

All NSAIDs work in basically the same way, so you might expect that patients would benefit from whichever NSAID they took. But actually, the way arthritis patients respond to an NSAID is individual: Quite often, patients who notice no improvement from one NSAID will do quite well when switched to another.

Sometimes patients must try several different NSAIDs before finding the right one: a drug that is both effective and does not cause side effects. As a general rule, if an NSAID is going to work for you it will be effective within seven to 14 days.

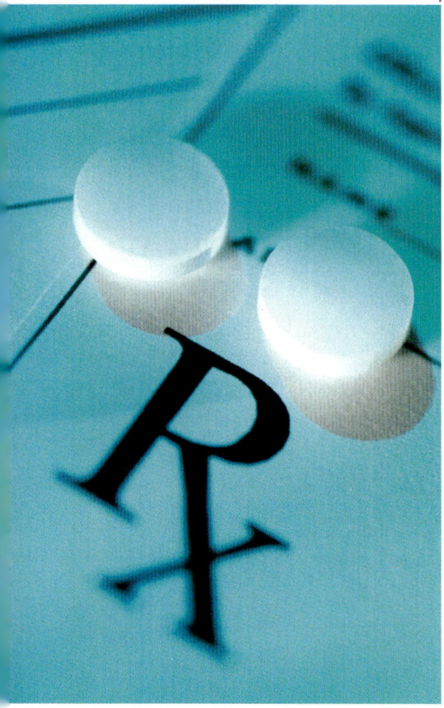

COX-2 Inhibitors: A Kinder, Gentler NSAID

The latest weapon in the pharmaceutical arsenal against arthritis pain is a new class of NSAID known as COX-2 inhibitors. Compared with the standard drugs used for arthritis pain and inflammation (ibuprofen, naproxen, aspirin, and others), these new prescription medications are less likely to cause bleeding and other gastrointestinal problems.

Aspirin: A New Role for an Old Standby

Aspirin remains a useful drug for occasional arthritis pain, but it has largely been replaced by newer NSAIDs in treating rheumatoid arthritis and other inflammatory types of the disease. Why? Greater irritation to the stomach lining and less convenience (an anti-inflammatory dose of aspirin requires taking four to six doses a day compared with only one or two daily doses of many other NSAIDs). But although its role in treating arthritis is fading, aspirin remains extremely useful for other purposes:

- It can significantly reduce the risk of heart attack and stroke, probably by reducing clot formation, when taken in low doses.
- Taking aspirin within 24 hours of a heart attack, and then daily for the next month, reduces the risk of dying from the heart attack by about 25 percent.
- It may help prevent memory loss in older people and slow down mental deterioration in people who are already senile.
- It may protect against colon cancer and may help in preventing other cancers as well.

That's especially good news for the estimated 30 percent of NSAID users who experience persistent gastrointestinal symptoms from those drugs and the 10 percent of users forced to discontinue taking NSAIDs because of side effects.

How it works. All NSAIDs relieve pain in the same basic way: by blocking an enzyme called cyclooxygenase, or COX. As discussed before, this enzyme produces prostaglandins, important chemicals that perform many different functions in the body.

Not until 1991 did researchers learn that COX comes in two forms: the "good" COX-1, which produces helpful prostaglandins that keep the gastrointestinal tract coated with protective mucus;

caution

People who need a COX-2 inhibitor but are allergic to sulfa drugs should avoid Celebrex, which can cause similar allergic reactions. Vioxx and Mobic don't cause such reactions.

and the "bad" COX-2, responsible for producing prostaglandins that play a big part in causing pain and inflammation in the body.

The standard NSAID takes a shotgun approach to the COX enzymes: It eases pain and inflammation by blocking COX-2, but unfortunately it also blocks COX-1, leaving your gastrointestinal tract susceptible to irritation that can cause ulcers and GI bleeding. Enter the COX-2 inhibitors, NSAIDs designed to affect only the COX-2 enzyme.

Hype from Reality

Celecoxib (Celebrex), the first COX-2 inhibitor, received federal approval in 1998. Rofecoxib (Vioxx) was approved in 1999. Additional COX-2 inhibitors are expected to hit the market in the near future. Although the COX-2's represent a major advance in arthritis treatment, keep these points in mind:

1. The many studies that have compared COX-2's with standard NSAIDs such as naproxen show that the COX -2's are no more effective against pain and inflammation than standard NSAIDs. If you are using a standard NSAID that works for you and is not causing problems, switching to one of the COX-2's won't do you much good.
2. Although COX-2's cause substantially fewer gastrointestinal side effects than standard NSAIDs, they are not risk-free. Clinical studies show that ulcers, irritation, and other problems still occur with COX-2's, although significantly less often than with standard NSAIDs.
3. The COX-2 inhibitors are much more expensive than standard NSAIDs.
4. Unlike aspirin, COX-2's don't prevent the blood from clotting, so they aren't helpful against heart attack and stroke. If you take COX-2's don't stop taking aspirin for your heart.

did you know

The COX-2 inhibitors Celebrex and Vioxx are no safer than standard NSAIDs when it comes to impairing kidney function in healthy older people, according to a July 2000 study in the *Annals of Internal Medicine*. If you're over 65 and regularly take Celebrex, Vioxx, or any other NSAID for arthritis, ask your doctor for a blood test to monitor your kidney function.

COX-2's and You: Perfect Together?

If you answer yes to one or more of the following questions, you may be a candidate for COX-2 therapy:

1. Do you have a previous or current history of ulcer disease?
2. Have you stopped using standard NSAIDs because you weren't able to tolerate them?
3. Are you older than 65? (Older people face an increased risk for bleeding and other gastrointestinal problems caused by standard NSAIDs.)
4. Are you currently taking a corticosteroid? (People taking prednisone or other corticosteroids are at increased risk for gastrointestinal bleeding.)

Different NSAIDs, Different Risks

NSAIDs cause more than 100,000 people to be hospitalized each year for problems such as gastrointestinal bleeding and ulcers. Studies have shown that some NSAIDs are more likely than others to cause serious problems.

Slight Risk

Celecoxib (Celebrex)
Etodolac (Lodine)
Ibuprofen (Motrin)
Meloxicam (Mobic)
Nabumetone (Relafen)
Rofecoxib (Vioxx)
Salsalate (Disalcid)

Moderate Risk

Diclofenac (Voltaren)
Ketoprofen (Orudis)
Oxaprozin (Daypro)
Naproxen (Naprosyn)
Tolmetin (Tolectin)

Serious Risk

Acetylsalicylic acid (Aspirin)*
Diflunisal (Dolobid)
Fenoprofen (Nalfon)
Indomethacin (Indocin)
Meclofenamate (Meclomen)
Piroxicam (Feldene)

*More than three 325 mg tablets daily

Mobic: A COX-2 Contender?

In April 2000, the FDA gave marketing approval to a new NSAID called Mobic (meloxicam). Mobic selectively inhibits COX-2 at therapeutic doses, but can't call itself a COX-2 inhibitor. As required by the FDA, drugs labeled as COX-2 inhibitors must target COX-2 exclusively even at twice their therapeutic dose, and Mobic doesn't meet that standard.

Comparison studies show that Mobic causes fewer side effects than standard NSAIDs. In addition, a daily dose of Mobic costs at least 20 percent less than Celebrex, Vioxx, Daypro, Relafen, and other expensive NSAIDs.

Visco-Supplementation: Help for the Knee-dy

If you have osteoarthritis of the knee and haven't been helped by acetaminophen or NSAIDs, you may want to consider a new procedure called visco-supplementation. It uses hyaluronic acid, a natural component of synovial fluid that helps to lubricate the knee and other joints.

In 1997, the FDA approved two visco-supplementation products for use in patients with knee pain caused by osteoarthritis: Synvisc (which requires three injections one week apart) and Hyalgan (five injections one week apart). The doctor numbs your skin with lidocaine and injects the jelly-like hyaluronic acid directly into the knee.

caution

Advertisements for Synvisc promote it as offering "drug-free relief for osteoarthritis knee pain." That claim is truthful in that Synvisc is technically classified as a medical device...but it somewhat misleadingly implies that Synvisc is a dietary supplement.

How it works. Once in the joint, it replaces the body's own hyaluronic acid that is lost when a joint is affected by osteoarthritis. Researchers have suggested several possible ways visco-supplementation may relieve knee pain, including bolstering the joint's shock-absorbing ability. Recent studies show that pain relief from visco-supplementation can last as long as 9 to 12 months and that the injections can be safely repeated.

BONING UP: Visco-supplementation is expensive. The cost of the medicine and three physician-administered injections is about $1,000. Since hyaluronic acid products are FDA-approved, insurance plans are likely to pay part or all of the cost of this therapy. But check with your individual insurance plan first.

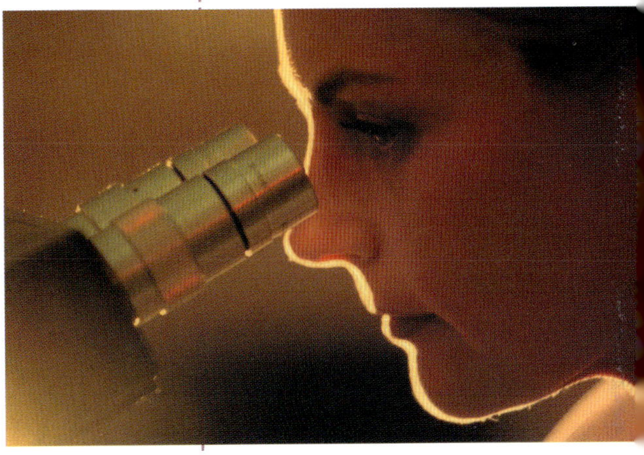

Visco-supplementation can undoubtedly help some patients, but rheumatologists seem to be taking a wait-and-see attitude toward the treatment. It may be especially useful for patients with OA of the knee who are not helped by NSAIDs or who cannot tolerate the drugs.

Side effects. They are usually mild: They include increased pain and swelling of the knee, as well as a rash and/or itching at the injection site.

Corticosteroids: Relief at a Price

The introduction of prednisone (a well-known cortisone derivative) in the 1950s revolutionized the treatment of RA. After patients took oral prednisone for a few days, their inflammation was quelled and their mobility restored.

But it didn't take long to discover the dark side of corticosteroids: the initial dose must be increased to maintain the benefits, which over time can cause serious side effects. Corticosteroids still remain one of the most effective of all treatments for patients with severe RA, although physicians try to use them as a last resort. One caution: Steroids should never be

Targeting the Joint

By injecting steroids directly into a painful joint, rheumatologists can greatly reduce the risk of serious complications that can occur when steroids are administered by mouth or by injection into muscles.

Minimizing infection. Anyone considering corticosteroid injections should weigh their temporary benefits against possible risks—particularly the risk of infecting the joint, which can be a serious matter. To minimize the risk of infection, physicians generally will not administer a steroid injection if the patient has an infection somewhere else in the body—a urinary or respiratory infection, for example.

taken orally by patients suffering from osteoarthritis, but they can be injected safely into the joint.

How they work. Some steroids are longer-acting with slower onset; others are shorter-acting with a quicker onset of symptom relief. Steroids seem to prevent the release of chemical-containing packets that tend to inflame and degrade cartilage and its supporting structures in the joint. New evidence suggests that corticosteroids also block cytokines, another class of chemicals responsible for inflammation.

BONING UP: **You should never abruptly stop taking corticosteroids. This can lead to a flare-up of symptoms. Instead you should be weaned from them gradually.**

A dramatic improvement. As treatments for RA, corticosteroids are either taken by mouth or injected into the muscle. Either way, they must be carefully administered, typically in "microdose" therapy: low-dose therapy that relieves inflammation while avoiding the serious side effects that higher doses can cause. In severe cases of RA, steroids can improve the disease dramatically, often producing a sense of well-being in the patient. But eventually, the drug stops working and side effects do occur.

A Point About Precautions

Serious side effects don't usually occur when corticosteroids are taken for only one or two months. Even in people who require large doses to control severe rheumatoid arthritis, many of the side effects will disappear after the medicine is stopped. Still you should be aware of them:

- Fluid retention. A person can gain 10 to 20 pounds, causing high blood pressure.
- Bone loss. Steroids can cause a loss of calcium from the bones, which can lead to osteoporosis and fractures of the back or other bones.
- Other side effects include cataracts; easy bruising of the skin; emotional changes; risk of infection; destruction of large joints, such as the hips; inhibition of growth in children.

did you know

To bring about prompt pain relief, rheumatologists often inject corticosteroids directly into sore joints of patients with RA, OA, or other types of arthritis. But repeated corticosteroid injections may damage cartilage, especially in weight-bearing joints such as the hip and knee. For this reason, injections into the same joint should usually be spaced at least four months apart.

DMARDs: Declaring War on RA

The NSAIDs have long been the mainstays of RA treatment, and for good reason: They are very effective in suppressing the hallmark of RA, inflammation—the destructive force that can lead to severe pain and joint damage. But in the past few years, RA treatment has expanded to include a new class of drugs, the disease-modifying antirheumatic drugs, or DMARDs.

Move over NSAIDs. The NSAIDs remain important in RA therapy, but rheumatologists no longer rely on them so heavily for several reasons:

- The high NSAID doses needed to relieve inflammation can sometimes cause serious complications.
- Experts realized that people with RA often experienced progressively worsening joint damage despite using pain-relieving NSAIDs.

- The DMARDs offer certain advantages over NSAIDs. DMARDs not only reduce inflammation but also slow down the joint destruction that, with NSAIDs, can continue even when inflammation has been quelled.

Once used only when other treatments had failed or only when joint damage became apparent, DMARDs are potent drugs that can have serious side effects. But in a major shift in the way RA is treated, many physicians now prescribe DMARDs as soon as RA is diagnosed, in an aggressive effort to halt the disease's progression and to prevent the damage it can cause to joints and internal organs.

The Older DMARDS: Still Effective After All These Years

Methotrexate

Used for decades to treat cancer and severe psoriasis, methotrexate became an RA drug when dermatologists prescribed it for psoriasis patients who also had RA—and noticed that their RA greatly improved. Use of methotrexate as a treatment for RA has soared since the early 1980s, and it now ranks as the most commonly prescribed DMARD.

caution

Since methotrexate can sometimes damage the liver, patients taking it should receive regular liver function tests—blood tests that can detect liver damage before it becomes severe.

How it works. RA occurs when the immune system mistakenly attacks the body's own joints, causing the chronic inflammation that can eventually destroy cartilage and bone. Like many DMARDs, methotrexate is an immunosuppressant, blunting the immune system's assault and thereby toning down RA's destructive and painful inflammation.

BONING UP: Methotrexate can lower your absorption of folic acid, causing a deficiency of this important vitamin. Some doctors recommend taking small daily doses of folic acid to prevent this potential shortfall.

Methotrexate is not only extremely effective for many RA patients, but also works faster than many other DMARDs, with improvement sometimes occurring within two weeks. It also has a good safety record: fewer than five percent of patients have to stop using it because of side effects. Methotrexate is usually given orally once a week.

Side effects. Since methotrexate can cause liver damage, patients need regular liver- function tests to check for damage—and must not drink alcohol heavily while taking the drug. Pregnant women should never take methotrexate because it may cause serious birth defects or even kill the fetus. The drug may also deplete sperm counts in men.

Gold

Gold therapy has been an important treatment for RA since the 1920s and remained a common option until methotrexate emerged in the 1980s. It can be administered either orally (given daily for an indefinite period of time) or by injection. The usual way is to inject it into the muscle weekly for four or five months. Maintenance injections are then given every two to four weeks indefinitely.

Oral gold (Ridaura) is easier to take and causes fewer side effects, but injectable gold is usually more effective. Some doctors begin with oral gold and, if no improvement is apparent, move on to injectable gold for six months.

How it works. Gold is slow-acting but helps to suppress joint inflammation, although experts are uncertain how it accomplishes that. Gold must be used for several months before improvement occurs. After using gold for two to four months, patients may notice reduced morning stiffness; joint inflammation along with pain and tenderness may start to diminish after four to six months.

Side effects. About 10 percent of children and adults on gold experience anemia, low white-blood-cell count, or liver-function test abnormalities. Gold can also harm the kidneys and cause a skin rash that disappears when the dosage is reduced.

Sulphasalazine

Developed in the 1930s, this drug is not widely used in the U.S. Impressive results from recent studies have sparked renewed interest in the drug, which works well for many RA patients

did you know

Patients with moderate to severe RA, and who can't tolerate or haven't responded to DMARD therapy, may be helped by undergoing a Prosorba column procedure. A coffee-mug-sized device approved by the FDA in March 1999, this new RA treatment apparently filters out antibodies and immune complexes that damage the joints of RA patients. Patients undergo 12 weekly outpatient sessions, each lasting about two hours. The cost of the treatments is now covered by Medicare.

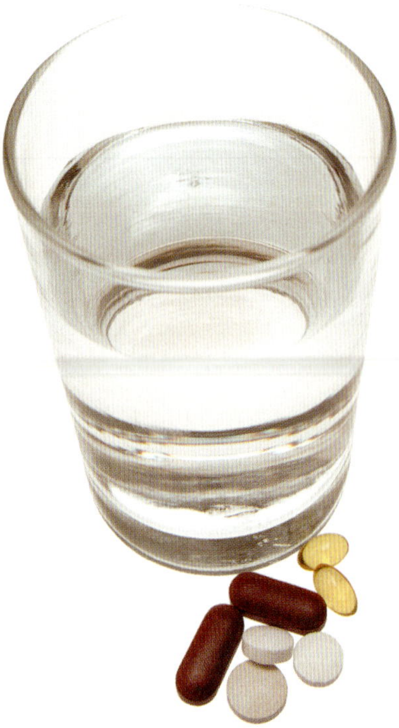

while rarely causing serious side effects. It seems to be quite effective when taken in combination with methotrexate.

How it works. Experts still don't know just how sulphasalazine works againt RA. Despite the drug's apparent effectiveness, the FDA has not yet approved it for use in treating RA. It is more widely used in Europe, mainly for pain relief and arthritis. Many U.S. rheumatologists prescribe it despite lack of governmental approval when other drugs have proven unsuccessful.

Side effects. The most common are nausea, headaches, dizziness, urine crystals, allergic reactions, or rashes. In rare cases, the drug can produce serious blood and liver toxicity.

Hydroxychloroquine

Long used as a treatment for malaria, hydroxychloroquine (brand name: Plaquenil) became an RA drug when malaria patients with RA noticed that it improved their arthritis. Hydroxychloroquine helps to relieve pain in many people with RA, but arthritis experts differ in their opinion of it: some recommend its use only after other drugs have failed, while others regard it as an effective drug that seldom causes side effects. It takes many months of treatment to show any benefit.

How it works. The medication is taken orally and almost always in combination with other drugs. Although experts are not sure exactly how it works, it can dramatically help some RA patients. Hydroxychloroquine, like methotrexate, can also reduce the dosage of corticosteroid (called a steroid-sparing effect) you would need to help relieve pain and inflammation.

Side effects. They include nausea, skin rashes, blood or protein in the urine, abnormal liver function, and injury to the back of the eye. Patients should have an eye examination every three to six months.

caution

People allergic to sulfa drugs should avoid sulphasalazine, which can cause serious adverse reactions.

Penicillamine

A synthetic offspring of penicillin, penicillamine is most effective for two kinds of patients—those with the specific genetic marker HLA-DR2 and those unresponsive to other DMARDs. Always taken with an NSAID or sometimes a steroid, penicillamine is considered a medication of last resort. On the other hand, some people with arthritis respond only to penicillamine.

How it works. Its effectiveness as an arthritis drug was discovered by accident. A chelating agent, penicillamine binds to heavy metals like gold and removes them from the body in patients. When it was used to treat gold overdosage in patients with RA, it relieved the arthritis. Penicillamine seems to act on the immune system in unknown ways to suppress the condition.

Side effects. Mild side effects include loss of taste as well as blood in the urine and abnormal liver function. On rare occasions, a muscular condition called myasthenia gravis can occur, causing a weakness of muscles. Patients should undergo regular blood and urine tests while taking the medication.

The Newest DMARDs

Etanercept

Revolutionary but extremely expensive, this new-generation DMARD was introduced in 1998. It is used to treat moderate to severe RA and is taken twice weekly by injection. Clinical trials found that etanercept (brand name: Enbrel) is both well tolerated and effective, decreasing pain and morning stiffness and reducing joint swelling and tenderness.

How it works. Etanercept is a "designer drug" specifically created to reduce levels of tumor necrosis factor (TNF), a protein produced by the immune system that seems to play a major role in causing both inflammation and joint damage in RA. (TNF has also been implicated in other chronic health problems, including inflammatory bowel disease and congestive heart failure.) Etanercept takes aim at TNF-alpha, the most notorious form of the protein.

In small doses, TNF plays a useful function in the body's immune response by helping cells repair themselves. But in RA and some other immune disorders, too much TNF is produced and it ends up destroying healthy tissue such as heart muscle (in congestive heart failure) and cartilage and bone (in RA).

what the studies show

In the August 1997 issue of *The Lancet*, 72 percent of patients who were given a corticosteroid (prednisolone), cytotoxin (methotrexate), and a DMARD (sulfasalazine) together showed improvement in their rheumatoid arthritis versus improvement in only 49 percent of the control group.

caution

Etanercept caused relatively few adverse effects in clinical trials. Nevertheless, some experts have expressed concern that the drug—by essentially shutting down part of the immune response—could increase patients' risk for lymphoma and other cancers.

In order to damage a cell, TNF must first latch onto "docking molecules" on the cell's surface called TNF receptors. Etanercept essentially consists of millions of man-made TNF receptors. When etanercept is injected into the bloodstream, these TNF receptors mop up the excess TNF alpha in the bloodstream, which prevents the protein from docking onto cells and causing an inflammatory response.

Help for the hopeless. Etanercept is considered a major breakthrough in the treatment of RA because it helps most patients who have failed to benefit from any other therapies. It has also been found effective when used in children suffering from the juvenile form of rheumatoid arthritis. Although etanercept is injected, it can be administered at home and is sold in prefilled syringes. (The drug must be kept refrigerated because it is a natural protein that can break down at room temperature.) At a yearly cost of about $12,000, etanercept is the most expensive of all treatments for RA.

Side effects. Some patients report mild reactions at the injection site and upper-respiratory-tract infections.

what the studies show

Multiple doses of infliximab combined with methotrexate can achieve long-term control of RA, according to a study in the April 2000 issue of *The Journal of Rheumatology*. In a study carried out on patients at three medical centers, the combination therapy effectively halted RA progression for up to 40 weeks. The majority of patients showed significant improvement after one or two weeks of treatment.

Infliximab

Approved as an RA treatment in 1999, this designer drug also knocks out tumor necrosis factor, but in a different way than etanercept. Infliximab (brand name: Remicade) consists of millions of identical antibodies, known as monoclonal antibodies, that have been synthesized specifically to target TNF alpha. Like etanercept, infliximab can produce dramatic improvement in RA patients who haven't responded to other therapies.

How it works. Just as the body's natural antibodies home in and destroy bacteria and viruses, infliximab's antibodies latch onto and inactivate TNF alpha. This greatly reduces the amount of TNF alpha available to inflame and damage the joints.

Infliximab is administered intravenously by a health-care professional—a procedure that takes about two hours and is given at 4-week or 8-week intervals. A year of treatment with infliximab costs about $10,000.

The Oral Tradition

If you don't like shots, you'll like the recently approved DMARD leflunomide (Arava), which can be taken orally, usually in 10-, 20-, or 100-mg tablets. In fact, it is typically prescribed in a "loading dose" of 100 mg daily for the first three days, then 20 mg daily afterward. (Patients who suffer side effects may have their dose lowered to 10 mg daily.)

How it works. Rather than focusing on TNF-alpha, like the newest DMARDs etanercept and infliximab, leflunomide works by disabling lymphocytes, white blood cells that play a role in the immune system's attack on the joints. It does the job by neutralizing an enzyme in the white cells. Studies show that leflunomide is at least as effective as methotrexate in slowing the progression of joint damage in RA patients. Equally promising, 40 to 60 percent of RA patients respond to this drug.

Side effects. Because leflunomide is new, no data exists on the potential long-term side effects. Your doctor should perform frequent lab tests, at least in the beginning of treatment, to monitor effects on the body.

Surgical Options That Make the Cut

Surgical procedures for OA and RA have clearly come a long way. Before the 1960s there wasn't much that surgery could do for osteoarthritis. The most common surgical procedure then was smoothing out irregular joint surfaces, as well as fusing a joint, which helped the pain but lead to other problems: Imagine trying to walk to the mailbox or up the stairs with a locked knee.

New joints and more. By far the greatest surgical advance in arthritis treatment is total replacement of an arthritic joint, a procedure known as total arthroplasty. Numerous joints can now

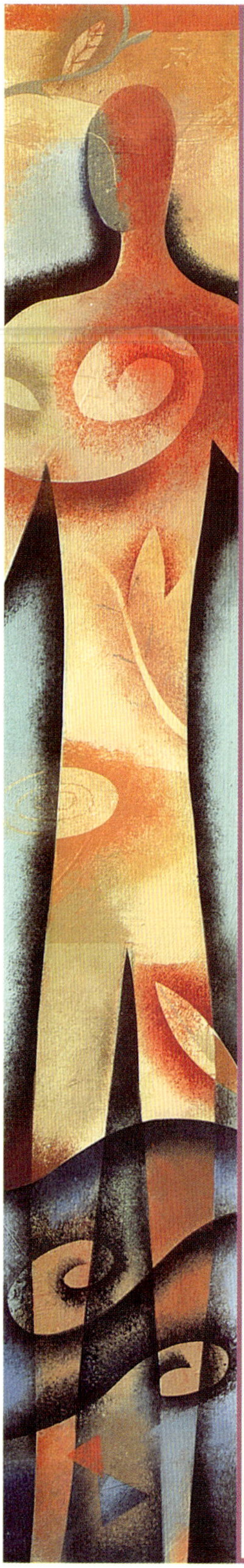

REAL-LIFE MEDICINE

Winning the Drug Wars

Fifty-five-year-old Gloria Baswell of Seattle, Washington, is all too knowledgeable about arthritis drugs: She has tried virtually all of them—and, until recently, found little benefit and many nasty side effects.

RA ran in Gloria's family: her mother had it and so did four first cousins on her mother's side of the family. Gloria developed a mild case of rheumatoid arthritis in her early 30s that mainly affected her knees and shoulders. But then, in 1987, Gloria's 19-year-old son was killed in a car accident and she was immersed in lawsuits.

"All the stress caused my RA to kick into overdrive," she says. "I woke up one morning and felt like someone had poured concrete into all my joints." Suddenly her fingers, wrists, elbows, shoulders, hips, knees, ankles, feet, toes, and even a joint in her neck were all affected.

So began nearly a decade of extreme pain and increasing disability. "It seemed that almost every day I was losing something else—the ability to brush my teeth, comb my hair, get out of bed, drive a car—all the things required to take care of myself," says Gloria, who was living in Gadsden, Alabama, at the time. A parade of doctors—first her family physician, then an orthopedist, then two successive rheumatologists—did what they could to help.

The doctors prescribed a total of more than 20 different nonsteroidal anti-inflammatory drugs to reduce Gloria's inflammation and pain. But, says Gloria, "I didn't get any real relief from any of them, just awful side effects, since the NSAIDs tore up my stomach, damaged my kidneys, and worsened my blood pressure."

Then there were the disease-modifying anti-rheumatic drugs, or DMARDs, which proved no more effective than the NSAIDs and even more toxic. "They put me on injectable gold salts, and I had a serious allergic reaction—difficulty breathing and a rash all over my body," Gloria recalls. The drug Plaquenil permanently damaged her distance vision. Her experiences were no better with other DMARDs, including methotrexate and sulphasalazine.

Finally Gloria was maintained on "tons and tons" of the steroid prednisone, administered both by mouth and injected into her joints. Gloria hated prednisone's side effects, which included weight gain and bloating, but it was the only drug that eased the inflammation and pain.

In 1995, Gloria underwent surgery on her left knee to remove synovial tissue that rubbed against her kneecap and prevented her from walking. "I was told that the surgery would last me about three years, and then I would need an artificial knee," says Gloria.

Then, in 1996, Gloria's rheumatologist told her about a clinical study being organized to test an experimental RA drug. It would be tested at several medical centers around the country, including the nearby University of Alabama at Birmingham. The study would be placebo-controlled, meaning some patients would get the real drug, others a sham treatment. Gloria signed up without hesitation. "We had tried everything," she explains, "and there was nothing else left for me."

Patients were told to inject themselves just under the skin twice a week. Gloria thought she noticed a lessening of pain and greater joint mobility soon after her first two injections. "But I knew it could be the placebo effect, so I reined in my excitement," says Gloria. Three weeks later there was no mistaking the improvement: Gloria felt better than at any time since she had developed RA. "I knew I'd found a miracle," she says.

"I knew I had found a miracle," says Gloria.

The drug Gloria was taking turned out to be etanercept (brand name Enbrel), one of several new drugs for treating RA. By binding to an inflammation-promoting substance known as tumor necrosis factor, etanercept can relieve pain and put a halt to joint damage.

In September 1998 Gloria paid her own way to Maryland to testify before an advisory committee considering whether etanercept should be approved by the FDA. "That was really one of the proudest days of my life, because I'm a shy person," says Gloria. "It was a huge room with cameras all over the place, since this was a breakthrough drug. But I told them my story and urged that they approve this drug for me and all the other people who were suffering the way that I was."

Etanercept received FDA approval in November 1998. In the four years Gloria has taken it, her RA has been in complete remission.

be replaced with artificial ones, including the shoulders, elbows, wrists, fingers, ankles, and toes. But the most common—and the most successful—joint replacement operations involve the hip and knee.

Each year in the U.S., some 120,000 hip-replacement and 150,000 knee-replacement operations are performed. The procedures relieve arthritis symptoms in knees and hips about 95 percent of the time—a much higher success rate than for any other commonly performed operation for arthritis. In the following pages, you'll find a laundry list of surgical options available to you.

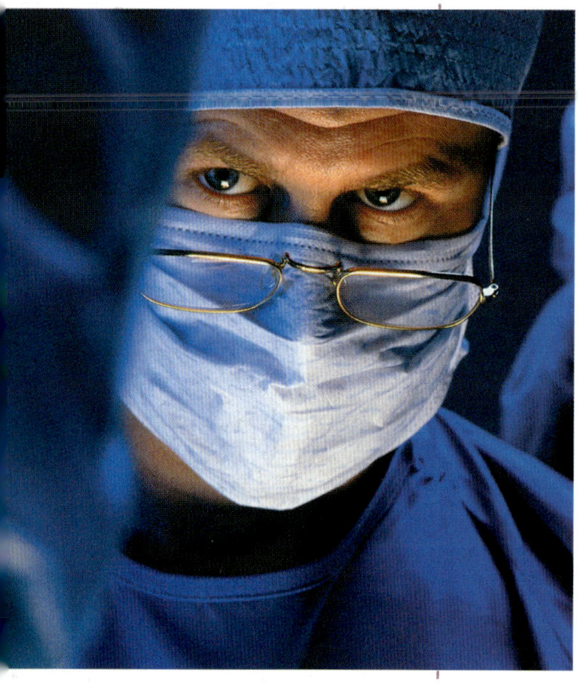

Is Surgery for You?

According to the Duke University Medical Center, you should ask yourself five questions to determine if you are a candidate for going under the knife:

1. Is your pain unacceptable?
2. Do you require narcotic pain relievers?
3. Have you tried all other options to achieve pain relief?
4. Are your goals realistic?
5. Are you in good physical condition?

If, after a great deal of thought, you decide to have surgery, selecting the right surgeon could be the most important decision you make. An orthopedic surgeon is a medical doctor with extensive training in diagnosing and surgically treating the musculoskeletal system, including bones, joints, ligaments, tendons, muscles, and nerves. Here are some ways to find the best surgeon out there:

- Ask your doctor for a referral. Just remember that doctors sometimes refer their friends in order to give them business, and many doctors are forced by HMOs to suggest surgeons on their HMO's list.

- Also call your local hospital, medical center, or medical society for referrals, or page through the book *The Best Doctors in America*, which is published annually.

- Call a teaching hospital for a referral. Teaching hospitals are often full of well-qualified surgeons who know about current procedures and practices. Remember, though, that if you decide on a teaching hospital, you probably shouldn't schedule your surgery in July, when most new trainees start their residencies and are at their least experienced.

Replacing Joints: Out with the Old, In with the New

For people with joints severely damaged by OA or RA, total joint-replacement surgery can be a godsend. The operation offers miraculous improvement for severely disabled people who would otherwise spend their lives bedridden or confined to a wheelchair.

The hip was the first joint to be replaced, in a procedure pioneered by Sir John Charnley of Great Britain in the 1960s. In this surgery, an entire joint is removed and replaced by an artificial joint made of durable plastic, metal, or ceramic. Thanks to improvements through the years, total hip and knee replacement are now highly successful operations with a failure rate of only one or two percent.

Now what? Patients typically return home four or five days after the surgery. Most are able to walk two to three months after hip surgery and about three months after knee replacement. (You should know that knee surgery causes more postoperative pain.) Full recovery from either hip or knee replacement surgery can take up to a year.

Surgical revisionism. All artificial joints wear out eventually. Fortunately, with today's newer materials and improved surgical techniques, most joints can be expected to last for 20 years or more. Joints wear out faster in younger people, whose higher activity levels put more stress and strain on them.

Replacing an artificial joint (a procedure known as revision arthroplasty) isn't as effective as the original: there is more pain and less freedom of movement. In fact, the eventual need for the second operation is a common argument for delaying the original surgery for as long as possible. On the other hand, the advice from some doctors—"put off your joint replacement until you can't stand the pain"—seems at odds with the mission of a patient who wants to take charge of his or her arthritis. Today's hip and knee replacement operations are almost always successful and consistently provide total or near-total relief from pain for many years.

what the studies show

A study in the April 2000 issue of *Bone and Joint Surgery* suggests that many people may not have to worry about undergoing a second hip-replacement operation. Researchers who followed up on hip replacements carried out between 1970 and 1972 found that 90 percent of the 327 hips replaced were still functioning up until the patient died or 25 years later for patients who were still alive. Today's hip replacements should last even longer, since they use a "cementless" technique that provides a firmer fit.

Interview with the Surgeon

When you have your short list of surgeons, here are some questions you should ask your prospective candidates:

- Are you board-certified?
- How many years have you been in practice?
- Do you receive any benefits or money from any orthopedic manufacturer?
- Will you be performing the joint procedure alone or with the assistance of a resident or fellow?
- Will you be in the operating room the entire time?
- How often is this surgery successful overall? How often when you perform it?
- How many of these surgeries have you performed? Over what period of time?
- How do the infection rates compare between this hospital and others in the area?
- How much pain will I experience and how will it be managed?

But Wait—There's More

If drugs or other nonsurgical treatments aren't helping you—but you don't yet need to replace a joint—you may find relief from several limited types of surgery.

Arthroscopy. This minimally invasive procedure, also known as "key hole" surgery, involves operating through small incisions in the skin. In arthritis treatment, arthroscopy is used mainly on knees. It can be quite effective in easing pain and stiffness, especially for people with a history of relatively mild knee symptoms that haven't improved with exercise, drugs, or other treatments. The procedure can be used to smooth out irregular cartilage surfaces, remove chunks of cartilage or bone spurs that have broken off and become loose in the knee joint, or trim away uneven edges of ligaments that fray or tear as OA progresses.

Arthroscopy can be performed under local anesthesia, and

patients generally go home the same day. Full recovery occurs in two to four weeks, sometimes even faster. Pain relief from arthroscopy typically lasts only two to three years—far briefer than that from total joint replacement surgery. But for those who can't afford the long convalescence that joint replacement requires, arthroscopy might be the ticket.

Osteotomy. Misalignments of the hip or knee bones can lead to OA or make it worse. Enter osteotomy—a surgical procedure that involves cutting wedges of bone from one or both of the weight-bearing bones of the joint, correcting the misalignment and shifting the body's weight on to the remaining healthy cartilage. Knee osteotomy requires only a day or two in the hospital; hip osteotomy requires a somewhat longer stay. Full recovery takes four to six months.

Osteotomy is most effective when the misalignment has caused cartilage to erode in just one area of the joint. The procedure usually can relieve symptoms for an average of about seven to 10 years. Osteotomies are especially helpful for very young, active patients with a crooked hip or knee. For them, osteotomy can help prevent OA or postpone the need for joint replacement until they're middle-aged or older.

Synovectomy. In this procedure—usually reserved for RA patients and mostly performed on the knee—surgeons remove inflamed synovium, the tissue that forms the inner lining of the joint. The synovium is the target of inflammation in RA, and removing it can prevent it from damaging the joint's cartilage and bone.

Another benefit of removing inflamed synovial tissue is a reduction in joint pain and inflammation. Unfortunately, synovectomy is not a permanent fix, since it is difficult to remove all the synovial tissue—and it can grow back.

Arthrodesis. Also known as joint fusion, this procedure is best done on smaller joints, such as fingers or toes, that have become damaged and unstable—usually because of RA. The joint is rendered permanently immobile through the use of metal screws or a special plaster, reducing pain. The procedure is especially successful on RA-affected wrists, relieving pain while still allowing good use of the hand. Ankles are another common site for joint-fusion surgery.

Forefoot reconstruction. This is one of the oldest and most effective surgical procedures for patients with RA—and one of the

did you know

Continuous passive motion, or CPM, can help the patient recover from joint-replacement surgery more quickly. A small machine actually moves the joint while a patient lies down or even sleeps. CPM has also been shown to help cartilage grow better after surgery. CPM can be used for up to eight hours per day for eight or more weeks.

Surgery Without the Glue

Hip replacements can now be performed without cement, especially in people under the age of 60 who have normal bones. The cementless parts of the artificial joint have a very bumpy surface, into which the patient's bones grow—anchoring it in place naturally.

A downside. The bones of some older patients suffering from osteoporosis may not be able to bond well with this kind of artificial joint because their bones are simply not strong enough.

few operations in which a good result is virtually guaranteed. It is performed when most or all of a patient's metatarsophalangeal joints (the ones connecting the toes to the foot) have become severely damaged due to RA. The surgeon excises the affected joints, leaving soft tissue where the joints were—but providing a surprisingly stable platform on which to walk.

New Surgical Procedures

Autologous chondrocyte implantation. Once cartilage is damaged, the injury is usually permanent. But a recently developed procedure called ACI is regenerating cartilage for some people with damaged knees.

How it works. First, a tiny chunk of cartilage, containing several thousand chondrocytes (cartilage-producing cells), is removed from the patient's healthy cartilage and sent to a laboratory where it is cultured in a petri dish. The cartilage cells are allowed to multiply until about 100 million are present.

The lab then freezes the cells and mails them back to the patient's physician, who reinserts the cartilage by opening the knee joint surgically and stitching or packing the new cartilage into the damaged area. After the knee is sewn back up, it is stabilized in a brace while the new cartilage takes hold. Since the implanted cartilage is the patient's own (i.e., autologous), there is no risk that the immune system will reject it.

Unfortunately, the procedure is very expensive (about $30,000), and so far it is intended only for repairing localized

did you know

There is some speculation that the success of ACI may be improved by rapidly transplanting the cultured chondrocytes into the defective cartilage. This can be done by culturing the cells in a location near the operating room, avoiding the delay of having the cells sent via the mail.

cartilage defects, although it may eventually prove useful for treating cartilage loss in OA.

Pain-Relief Strategies: Try the Golden Oldies

Amid all the dramatic news about arthritis breakthroughs, people may tend to overlook some of the older, simpler but nonetheless helpful treatments available for osteoarthritis and rheumatoid arthritis. Foremost among these old but often-helpful standbys are heat, cold, and topical rubs.

Heat or Cold? Knowing When to Use What

Many people with arthritis can achieve temporary pain relief by using heat or cold. Heat works better for relaxing muscles and for soothing chronic aches and pain, while cold is the better treatment when joints are acutely swollen or inflamed.

Some joints like it hot. Heat helps to stimulate blood circulation and is a great way to relax stiff muscles or muscle spasms and soothe aching joints. People generally find more joint-pain relief with moist heat than with dry—probably because moist heat does a better job of warming the tissues underlying the skin. Moist heat in the form of a hot bath is surely one of the oldest of all treatments for arthritis.

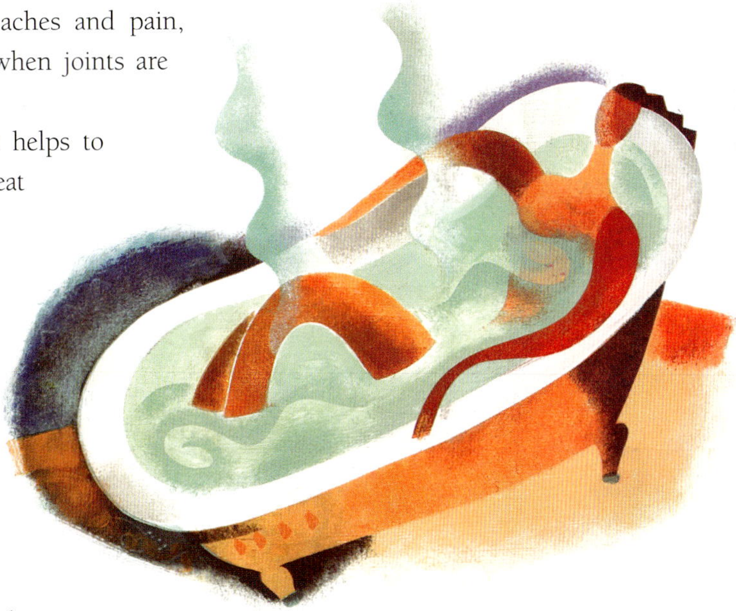

Ordinary superficial heat—the kind produced by a warm bath or a heating pad—works best for joints closer to the skin surface such as the knuckles and other joints of the hands. For this reason, people with OA of the hands may find significant pain relief by immersing their hands in hot water or using heated mittens.

Tips for Using Heat and Cold

- You can use heat or cold several times during the day, but don't apply either one to an area for more than 15 or 20 minutes at a time.
- Be sure to put a towel or some other barrier between your skin and the cold or heat source.
- Never use heat treatment together with Ben-Gay, Aspercreme, or any other topical pain-relief product, since the combination could cause a burn.
- Since any form of heat can potentially cause burns, people with diabetes, poor circulation, or any other health problem that impairs sensation should be especially careful not to overuse heat.
- Check your skin regularly when using heat or cold to prevent frostbite or burns.
- When using a heating pad, stick to the low and medium settings and avoid "high."

Getting heat to reach deeper joints, such as the hip or knee, requires use of diathermy, in which heat is generated by devices that emit shortwave, microwave, or ultrasound radiation. (Ultrasound penetrates more deeply than microwave or short-wave radiation.) Diathermy treatments are usually available only in a physician's office or in clinics and can be expensive.

The comforts of a cooldown. Cold is better than heat for joints that are acutely painful or inflamed—perfect for pain caused by rheumatoid arthritis. Applying cold can be useful after exercise, since it can reduce the swelling and muscle ache that may follow a strenuous workout.

How it works. Cold has both anti-inflammatory and pain-relieving properties. It can help numb a painful area, and by reducing the swelling that interferes with healing, can speed up recovery from "overuse injuries" such as tennis elbow or shin splints.

You can quickly make an ice pack by filling a small zip-lock plastic bag with ice. If ice isn't handy, you can improvise by wrapping a bag of frozen vegetables or a cold can of soda in a towel and applying your "veggie" or "cola" pack to a painful joint.

Running hot and cold. Some people find that alternating heat and cold treatments provides better relief for arthritis pain than using either of them alone. For example, you can apply a heating pad for three or four minutes, let your joint rest for minute, and apply an ice pack for one minute. Then repeat the cycle several times...trying to end the routine with warmth.

Topical Pain Relievers: What's the Rub

What if you could rub aspirin or other NSAIDs directly into a painful joint without having to swallow a tablet or capsule? Ideally, you would get the same pain relief that NSAIDs provide—but without the stomach irritation they can cause.

Such topical drugs are technically known as rubefacients. They may indeed provide temporary but noticeable pain relief with much less risk of encountering the sometimes serious side effects that oral NSAIDs can cause.

The salicylate products. You're probably familiar with several topical pain relievers, including Ben-Gay, Aspercreme, and Myoflex. They and some 40 other nonprescription products contain salicylates, a family of drugs that reduces pain and inflammation and that includes acetylsalicylic acid, the active ingredient in aspirin.

How they work. Rub-on salicylates are used not only for minor arthritis pain (usually the fingers, knuckles, elbows, and knees) but also for strains, sprains, tendinitis, and sports injuries. The two main ingredients are methyl salicylate (contained in Ben-Gay) and trolamine salicylate (the ingredient in Aspercreme and Myoflex) and are usually applied one to three times per day. They may relieve pain in several possible ways:

- When rubbed on, salicylates travel a short distance (about three or four millimeters) below the skin, perhaps far enough for some of the ingredient to penetrate directly into a sore joint.

- When salicylates are rubbed on the skin, measurable amounts are absorbed into the bloodstream and may reach

did you know

In the late 1800's, the Parisian physician Dr. Bengue dispensed pills and ointments to arthritis patients. One of his ointments, Baum Bengue, contained a combination of methyl salicylate and menthol. The same ingredients are still used in the ointment's modern-day version, now called Ben-Gay.

Plug In to a Stimulating Therapy

Electrical stimulation is the application of small doses of electricity to painful joints and supporting structures. If you like medical jargon, it is officially known as transcutaneous electrical nerve stimulation, or TENS for short.

How it works. Electrodes are coated with a gel and attached to the skin on or near the affected area. The electrodes are attached by wires to the TENS unit, which sends low-level electricity into the skin (using a nine-volt battery) through the wires and electrodes. Patients may feel a tingling sensation or nothing at all.

Does it work? Clinical studies in treating arthritis pain have yielded conflicting results. In RA patients, studies show that TENS can reduce pain and improve flexibility; in OA patients, the results are mixed.

Pain relief from TENS may last only as long as the treatment or for several hours afterward. One advantage: Patients can use TENS therapy at home after they have been instructed in its use. A caution, though: People with cardiac pacemakers should never use a TENS unit since the electrical impulses could interfere with the pacemaker's function.

the joint that way. In one study, subjects were asked to rub a methyl salicylate product on a large joint four times a day. Researchers found that the equivalent of two aspirin tablets was absorbed into the bloodstream.

- Ads for Ben-Gay, for example, boast that it "has warming power that penetrates deep down." Some experts contend that this warming sensation accounts for the product's effectiveness by distracting users from their joint pain.

Capsaicin products. The other main class of topical products for arthritis pain contains capsaicin (pronounced cap-SAY-shun), the chemical responsible for the "hotness" of red pepper and cayenne. Many nonprescription creams are available that contain 0.025 to 0.075 percent capsaicin; examples include Capzaisin P, Zostrix, Zostrix HP, and Absorbine Arthritis Strength. (Capsaicin products are also used for other painful conditions, including shingles and post-mastectomy pain.)

How they work. Most experts believe capsaicin products are more effective than salicylates in relieving minor arthritis pain. One reason: Experts have a clearer idea of how capsaicin works. It appears to dull pain by "robbing" sensory neurons (the nerves that signal pain, touch, and other sensations) of substance P—a chemical responsible for transmitting the pain felt in various arthritic conditions to the brain. In addition, capsaicin may trigger the release of endorphins, the body's natural pain relievers.

> **caution**
>
> Apply capsaicin cream with a plastic glove to minimize contact with the skin, and keep it away from the eyes and other sensitive tissues. Also, never use capsaicin products on broken or irritated skin or in combination with a heating pad.

Capsaicin is considered particularly useful against OA of the fingers, wrists, hands, and knees. But to be effective, capsaicin products must be applied frequently—four times a day. People generally notice improvement after applying capsaicin cream for three to seven days. For the first seven to 10 days of use, you may feel significant stinging or burning that usually fades after a week or two of regular use.

> **BONING UP:** **Capsaicin takes at least a few days and as much as a month before its effect really kicks in. This delay in relief may be due to the time it takes to deplete substance P from nerve endings.**

One drawback to long-term use of capsaicin products is their expense. At a nearby pharmacy, a two-ounce tube of Ben-Gay cost $5.99 compared with $20.99 for a two-ounce tube of Zostrix H-P.

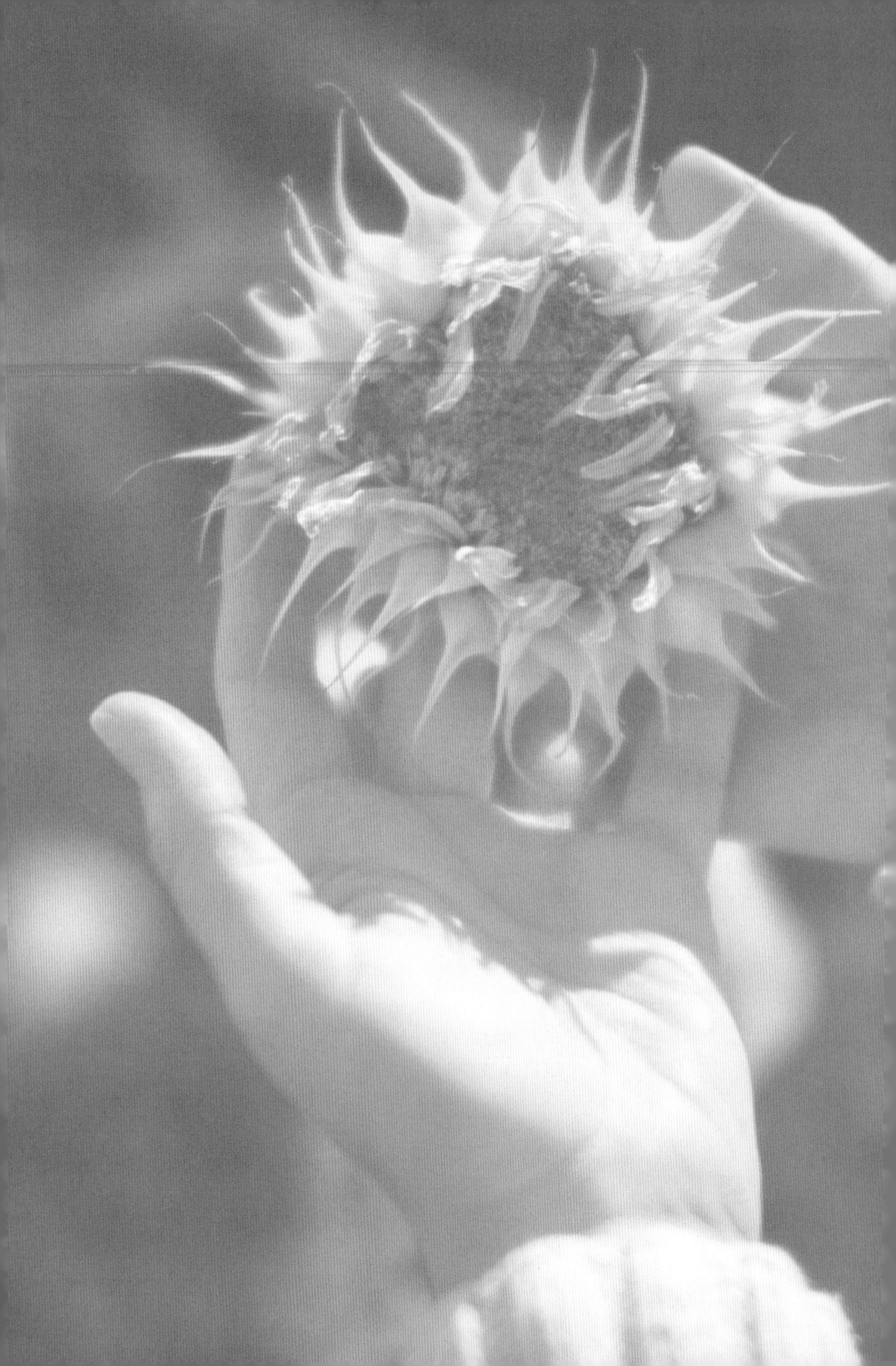

6 Treating Arthritis: Alternative Therapies

Most arthritis patients resort to a nonconventional remedy at least once. And for people who want to take charge of their arthritis, opting for alternative therapies has obvious attractions. But be cautious: alternative medicine can imperil as well as empower.

KEY CONCEPT

Alternative therapies offer self-empowered patients another avenue to gain control of their disease. Always weigh the evidence of a therapy before giving it a try.

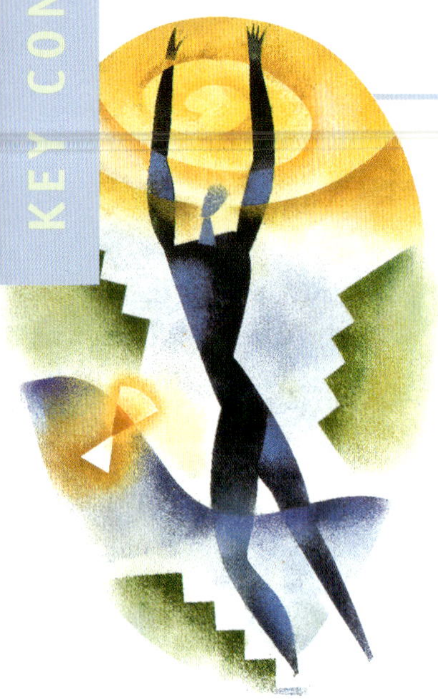

Alternative Goes Mainstream

Once they were exiled to the fringes of medicine, but alternative therapies are now a major part of its fabric. Consider these findings from a large nationally representative telephone survey published in the *Journal of the American Medical Association* in 1998:

- During 1997, more than four out of 10 Americans—some 83 million people—had used at least one alternative therapy.
- Visits to alternative medicine practitioners increased by nearly 50 percent between 1990 and 1997.
- The number of visits to alternative practitioners during 1997 totaled 629 million—exceeding the total visits to all U.S. primary-care physicians.
- Americans spent $5.1 billion for herbal products in 1997.

Alternatives and arthritis. Many arthritis patients have eagerly embraced alternative therapies. One recent survey concluded that two-thirds of them have at least experimented with alternative remedies, and many use such treatments regularly. And there are certainly a lot to choose from.

Boning Up: Use alternative therapies to supplement rather than replace standard treatments such as prescription drugs, weight loss, and exercise.

Hundreds of alternative treatments have been promoted for treating arthritis, most of them herbs and other dietary supplements. Unfortunately, just a handful of these remedies have been studied thoroughly enough to determine whether they are safe and effective.

Proceed with Caution

Many arthritis patients have been victimized by remedies that promised the moon but succeeded only in depleting their wallets and, in some cases, endangering their health. By following these guidelines, you can help ensure that alternative treatments won't create more problems than the symptoms you are trying to vanquish.

- Since symptoms of arthritis wax and wane, be careful about crediting an alternative remedy for improvements that might have occurred anyway.
- Just because herbs and other alternative remedies are "natural" does not mean they're harmless. After all, about one-fourth of today's prescription drugs were originally isolated from plants. Herbs can be potent drugs, and you should stop using them or consult your doctor if side effects occur. Better yet, tell your doctor about the herb before you take it. Interactions can occur with a drug you are already taking.
- Don't assume that the ingredients listed on dietary-supplement labels are actually present. Manufacturers are under no obligation to guarantee the identity and quality of their products.
- Avoid any alternative therapies that are supported only by testimonials—you owe it to your health to make sure that claims can be supported by scientific research.
- If you're pregnant or nursing, check with your doctor before taking a dietary supplement for arthritis.
- Beware of alternative therapists who claim to possess "secret" knowledge or cures—ethical practitioners don't deal in secrets.

This chapter offers guidance to those arthritis patients who want to use the most promising alternative treatments wisely and effectively. The focus is mainly on treatments that are currently "hot" (glucosamine, chondroitin sulfate, and SAM-e, for example), widely used by arthritis patients (acupuncture and chiropractic), especially promising (collagen II supplements for rheumatoid arthritis), or widely recognized as arthritis alternatives (copper bracelets and DMSO).

Hands-On Therapies: Good for Body and Mood

The laying on of hands can help relieve musculoskeletal pain and emotional distress—a natural consequence of managing a chronic disease like arthritis. With any form of bodywork, success depends on the training, skill, and experience of the practitioner. If there is no improvement, try another technique or practitioner.

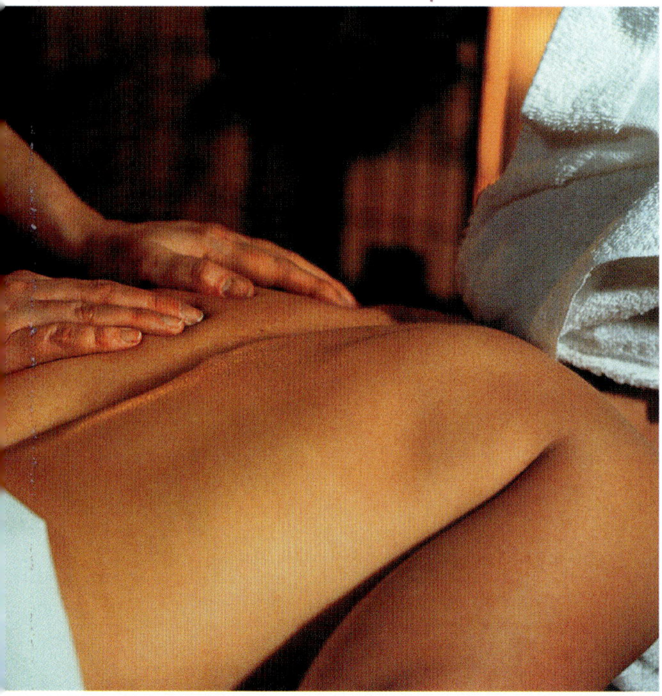

Massage: Touch Therapy

The first written references to massage date to about 2000 B.C.—but in all likelihood, its use probably extends back to prehistory. One proponent of massage therapy was Hippocrates, who believed that the therapy restored the body's nutritive fluids to their natural free movement.

How it works. For people with arthritis, massage therapy can help in several ways. It relaxes muscles and decreases muscle stiffness and spasm; it decreases pain; and it increases the range of motion of the joints. (Interestingly, research has shown that one of the benefits long claimed for massage—increased blood flow to the muscles—actually doesn't occur.)

Anyone seeking massage therapy (also known as bodywork) can choose from more than 100 different types, ranging from gentle touching like the Alexander technique to deep-massage techniques such as rolfing and neuromuscular massage.

> "There are few people who would dispute the short-term benefits of massage, especially for pain relief."
>
> —J.J. Fiechtner, M.D., M.P.H. and R.R. Brodeur, D.C., Ph.D., Rheumatology Disease Clinics of North America

Massage therapy can be administered by massage therapists (most of whom are trained in many of these techniques) as well as physical therapists, chiropractors, and physicians. Or, as someone determined to take charge of your arthritis, you can take things into your own hands (see *Do-It-Yourself Massage*, next page).

BONING UP: Look for a state-licensed massage therapist, since amateurs may do harm. Insurance and managed care plans may pay for massage when recommended by your physician.

A Bodywork Menu

There is more than one way to decrease pain and relax muscles. Here is an a la carte list of some bodywork approaches:

Neuromuscular therapy (NMT) uses precisely focused, calibrated pressure to relax areas of tension or pain that may be contributing to pain in other parts of the body, and ease tense muscles that may be pulling joints out of position. Like physical therapists, competent NMT practitioners should possess a thorough knowledge of human anatomy and be able to recommend therapeutic exercises.

Rolfing is similar to NMT. Its goal is to normalize posture and joint function by relaxing muscles that are tight and contracted. However, there is a difference: Rolfing focuses on loosening muscles and connective tissues that have adhered to bone structures.

Shiatsu uses focused finger pressure to ease pain and stiffness. Like acupuncture and acupressure, it is based on the belief that the fingers can direct therapeutic energy to ailing tissues and organs.

Do-It-Yourself Massage

Self-massage may not be as satisfying as the laying on of hands done by a professional, but it can make you feel better. Tense muscles can aggravate arthritis pain, and kneading the muscles—especially the ones around sore joints—can help. Muscles in the neck, arms, fingers, shoulders, thighs, and legs are all accessible to self-massagers. Here are some tips for doing your own bodywork:

- Apply baby powder or baby oil to the area before massaging; it helps reduce friction and facilitates working your muscles.
- Try a variety of different movements, including firm stroking with the palm and fingers, kneading (by "cupping" muscles between the palm and fingers or squeezing with the thumb and fingers), and making circles with the heel of your hand or your fingertips.
- Don't massage the same spot for more than about 15 or 20 seconds.
- A vibrating massager may be useful for areas that are not easily accessible.
- Don't massage a joint that is severely inflamed or where the skin is irritated, and stop if the massage causes pain.

Feldenkrais practitioners teach people how to walk, sit, and work in ways that help restore joint-friendly posture and balance.

Yoga can help improve range of motion and strengthen muscles around joints. In one clinical trial, 17 people with OA of the hands used yoga to help relieve pain. Compared with patients who did no yoga, those who practiced it ended the experiment with less pain and greater range of motion in afflicted joints.

Manipulation: Pain Relief with a Twist

Manipulation involves twisting, thrusting, or pressing of the body. The treatment can help to relieve some types of pain, and it works better than stretching to increase the joint's range of motion.

Several types of health-care professionals use manipulation in their practice, including osteopaths, physical therapists and—most notably—chiropractors, who emphasize manipulation of the spine. With their focus on drugless healing and wellness, chiropractors have profited from the public's surging interest in alternative medicine.

The national telephone survey cited earlier found that chiropractors were by far the most popular alternative practitioners, accounting for more than 30 percent of all visits to alternative therapists in 1997; for the survey's arthritis patients in particular, chiropractic along with relaxation were the therapies they used most often. But does spinal manipulation—by chiropractors or anyone else—actually help in treating arthritis?

Some two dozen controlled clinical studies have investigated spinal manipulation for a variety of health problems, not including osteoarthritis. So far, spinal manipulation has been found effective for treating one condition: common acute low-back pain that has lasted for three weeks or less. In addition, recent research suggests that the therapy may be helpful against neck pain.

How it works. Treatment for back or neck pain is the main reason that people see chiropractors. But to the chiropractic

what the studies show

In its May 2000 issue, *Consumer Reports* published results of its survey of more than 46,000 readers on their use of alternative therapies—the largest such study ever conducted. Among readers with arthritis who had received chiropractic care, some 25 percent reported feeling "much better" from the treatment, while nearly 40 percent said chiropractic care had "helped only a little or not at all."

Chiropractic Do's and Don'ts

If you decide to see a chiropractor keep the following in mind:

- Be wary of claims that spinal manipulation can treat health problems in other parts of the body.
- Manipulation is a forceful procedure that—especially when it involves the neck—carries with it a very small but finite risk of injury, including stroke or paralysis. People with arthritis or ankylosing spondylitis should never undergo manipulation of the neck.
- Be skeptical of the need for long-term treatment. The main benefit of manipulation is rapid relief from low-back pain. If you haven't noticed significant improvement after three weeks of treatment, it's unlikely that manipulation will help you.

profession, manipulating the spine can have an impact on the entire body. Chiropractic theory is based on the notion that small spinal misalignments, known as subluxations, are the cause of numerous health problems ranging from hypertension to ear infections. Chiropractors contend that spinal manipulations (which they call "adjustments") can correct those misalignments and thereby clear up health problems or, when done regularly, prevent them from occurring. But despite researchers' efforts to pinpoint them, subluxations remain entirely theoretical.

The bottom line. Spinal manipulation is a useful therapy for acute low-back pain and possibly for neck pain, but its effectiveness for relieving back pain due to osteoarthritis remains to be proven.

Acupuncture: Treatment with a Point

A part of the health-care system of China, acupuncture has been used for more than 2,500 years. It involves stimulating certain points on or just under the skin by inserting very thin needles and then "manipulating" them, either manually or with electric current.

How it works. Acupuncture is based on the idea that an essential life force, known as *qi*, flows through the body along several channels, or meridians. Disease occurs when one or more of these channels becomes blocked. Inserting needles at appropriate sites—the acupuncture points—along the affected channels restores health by enabling *qi* to flow freely again.

BONING UP: **Similar to acupuncture, acupressure uses fingertip pressure instead of needles to help disperse lactic acid that builds up in muscles. It is a safe technique that you can learn and use on yourself.**

Acupuncture was unknown to most Americans until President Nixon's visit to China in 1972. Since then, interest in acupuncture has surged, and the therapy is now widely used in chronic pain programs and clinics in the U.S.

More than one million Americans undergo acupuncture treatment each year—a large proportion of them patients with arthritis and other painful musculoskeletal problems. Surveys of rheumatology patients who consult alternative-medicine practitioners show that acupuncture is the therapy they use most often.

Considering the controversy. Despite its popularity, acupuncture remains controversial. Many Western physicians contend that acupuncture has no rational basis, since the meridians it acts upon have never been detected. Acupuncture's effectiveness, they say, can be explained by the placebo effect (patients' expectation that a treatment will work) or by distraction (diverting patients' attention from their symptoms by irritating or stimulating another part of the body).

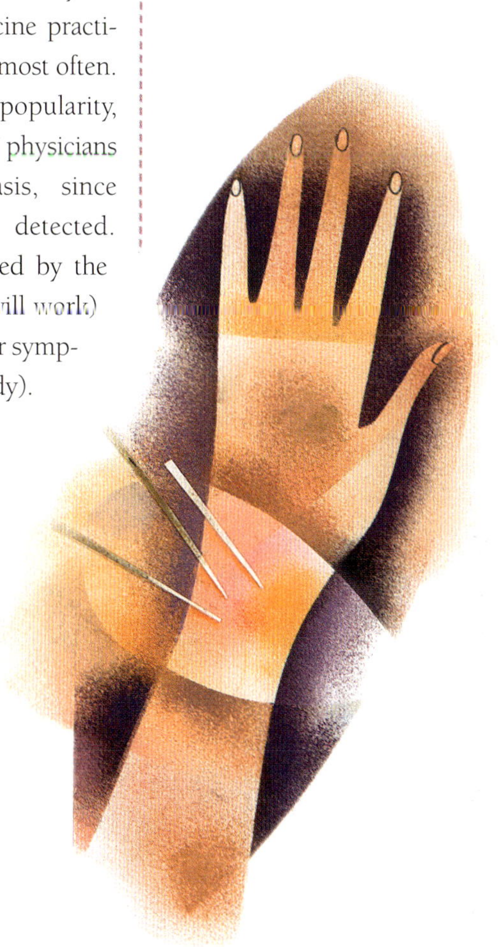

Acupuncture received a major boost in 1997, when a panel of experts convened by the National Institutes of Health evaluated hundreds of studies on acupuncture. Their conclusion: Acupuncture was effective for certain medical conditions—postoperative dental pain and nausea and vomiting associated with chemotherapy—and showed promise against a number of others, including several problems affecting the muscles and joints.

The panel cited evidence that acupuncture can trigger biological effects that may explain the benefits observed in many studies and by many patients. "Considerable evidence" suggests that painkilling chemicals called endorphins are released during acupuncture, and studies also show that acupuncture can alter immune function, the panel concluded.

When Does It Work Best

Fibromyalgia and tennis elbow were singled out as musculoskeletal problems that might be especially amenable to acupuncture. The panel noted that these problems were often treated with NSAIDs or steroid injections; both treatments can cause "deleterious side effects," the panel stated, and evidence supporting their use "is no better than that for acupuncture."

> **"The data in support of acupuncture are as strong as those for many Western medical therapies. One of the advantages of acupuncture is that the incidence of adverse effects is substantially lower than that of many drugs or other accepted medical procedures used for the same conditions."**
>
> —NIH Consensus Development Panel on Acupuncture, 1997

As for acupuncture's effectiveness against osteoarthritis, the NIH panel found the evidence "less convincing." Nevertheless, it noted that some clinical trials involving acupuncture and osteoarthritis have shown "positive" results.

caution

Improperly administered acupuncture has caused serious complications, including life-threatening infections, nerve damage, and puncture of internal organs, including the lungs. Look for a practitioner who is experienced and uses sterilized, disposable needles. Contact the American Academy of Medical Acupuncture (800-521-2262; www.medical-acupuncture.org) for a list of physicians trained in acupuncture. Other practitioners (mostly nonphysicians) have met standards for safety and experience set by the National Certification Commission for Acupuncture and Oriental Medicine; for a list, contact the commission at 703-548-9004; www.nccaom.org.

The bottom line. Acupuncture has shown particular promise in treating fibromyalgia. People with osteoarthritis and other forms of arthritis may also want to try acupuncture, especially if other treatments haven't helped. Repeat visits will probably be needed, and they can be expensive: The first visit typically costs $75 to $150, with subsequent ones costing $35 and up. If you don't notice improvement in your condition after six treatments, then the therapy is probably not going to work for you.

Dietary Supplements: Therapy You Can Swallow?

Supplements for treating arthritis and other health problems have soared in popularity in recent years, thanks largely to a federal law, the 1994 Dietary Supplement Health and Education Act. Although some of the supplements have helped arthritis patients, this law essentially eliminated FDA oversight of all dietary supplements—with unfortunate consequences for consumers.

Thanks to the 1994 law, makers of dietary supplements are not obligated to show that their products are safe or effective—

the essential standards that all drugs must meet. The FDA can act to remove a supplement from the market only if it can show that well-documented health problems are associated with its use. Furthermore, manufacturers have no obligation to ensure that the ingredients they list on their label are actually in the product or are present in the amount claimed.

> **"We all take for granted that because a product says that something's in it on the label, it's actually in the bottle. That's not the case with dietary supplements."**
>
> **—Dr. David Kessler, former FDA commissioner**

Choose wisely. Faced with this wild-west situation, you need to tread carefully when buying dietary supplements. To improve the odds that the products you buy will actually work and will be safe to use, buy supplements from large manufacturers that distribute their products nationally. Studies that have analyzed dietary supplements suggest that bigger companies generally do a better job of quality control than smaller firms.

For every supplement ingredient that shows promise against arthritis, there may be dozens of brands that offer it. If possible, find out the particular brands used in the studies that have helped create enthusiasm for the supplement—and buy that one. As we note below, for example, only one of the numerous glucosamine/chondroitin sulfate products on the market has a clinical-trial track record.

Glucosamine and Chondroitin Sulfate: Hope in a Bottle

The dietary supplements glucosamine and chondroitin sulfate became famous almost overnight in 1997, when they were touted in *The Arthritis Cure*. This best-selling book described some 30 published clinical studies—mainly from Europe—that found that glucosamine (made from crab shells) or chondroitin (made mainly from cow tracheas) help against osteoarthritis.

Promising research. The studies generally showed that glucosamine or chondroitin sulfate works significantly better than placebos in relieving pain and improving the mobility of osteoarthritis patients. In addition, the supplements worked at least as well as nonsteroidal anti-inflammatory drugs such as ibuprofen (Advil, Motrin IB), and each appeared quite safe, with very few side effects observed.

on the horizon

A federally sponsored study will investigate glucosamine and chondroitin sulfate as treatments for OA of the knee. Sponsored by the National Institutes of Health, the $6.6 million double-blind, placebo-controlled study will involve more than 1,200 patients and be carried out at several medical centers around the U.S. Patients will be randomly assigned to take either glucosamine, chondroitin sulfate, a combination of glucosamine and chondroitin sulfate, a nonsteroidal anti-inflammatory drug, or a placebo. The study is expected to begin in 2001.

A Consumer's Guide: What You Should Know Before Taking It

- Studies show that it typically takes a month before users of glucosamine and chondroitin sulfate notice any benefit versus one or two weeks for NSAIDs. If you don't notice improvement after about two months, these supplements probably aren't for you.
- When buying glucosamine, choose the "hydrochloride" form over the "sulfate" form. A typical 500 mg capsule of glucosamine sulfate contains only 239 mg of glucosamine versus 407 mg of glucosamine in a 500-mg capsule of glucosamine hydrochloride.
- Most of the clinical trials involving glucosamine and chondroitin sulfate used daily doses of 1,200 mg of chondroitin sulfate and 1,500 mg of glucosamine.
- Diabetics may want to avoid glucosamine or have their blood-sugar levels tested more frequently because animal studies have suggested that glucosamine may worsen insulin resistance.
- People who have a bleeding disorder or are taking a blood thinner should be aware that chondroitin sulfate also acts as a blood thinner.

did you know

U.S. sales of products containing glucosamine and/or chondroitin sulfate totaled more than $1.2 billion in 1999.

NSAIDs and other drugs currently used to treat OA can only help relieve symptoms—and the NSAIDs in particular can cause serious side effects, especially when taken for long periods of time. That explains the interest in glucosamine and chondroitin sulfate, which seem to be just as effective as certain NSAIDs but much safer.

How they work. When glucosamine and chondroitin sulfate are swallowed, they are absorbed into the bloodstream and work their biochemical benefits in the joints. It's still not clear just how these two supplements relieve the symptoms of OA, but evidence suggests that they may slow the progression of cartilage loss—and may even help rebuild cartilage that has started to break down.

In the joints of the human body, glucosamine and chondroitin sulfate are important building blocks of cartilage—particularly of the proteoglycans, the large molecules that give cartilage its resilience. Taking glucosamine as a dietary supplement appears to combat osteoarthritis by stimulating the chondrocytes (cells that manufacture cartilage) to produce more cartilage; chondroitin sulfate seems to help against osteoarthritis by interfering with enzymes that degrade cartilage.

Glucosamine and chondroitin sulfate can be purchased individually or as combination glucosamine/chondroitin supplements (brands include Cosamin DS, Osteo Bi-Flex and Natural Pain Relief Formula). Although combinations should theoretically be more useful than single-ingredient products, most of the clinical trials have tested glucosamine or chondroitin individually rather than in combination.

So far, all the studies carried out in the U.S. on glucosamine combined with chondroitin have involved one brand, Cosamin DS. Results of two placebo-controlled clinical trials were recently reported—one involving 34 male U.S. Navy Seals with osteoarthritis of the knee or lower back, the other involving 100 patients with OA of the knee. In both studies, patients taking the supplements generally experienced more pain relief than patients in the placebo group.

The bottom line. Both glucosamine and chondroitin sulfate show promise in treating OA. More studies are needed to prove their effectiveness, but they do seem to relieve the symptoms of OA while posing relatively few risks. Since they don't seem to interact with other OA drugs such as NSAIDs, they may allow you to cut back on the NSAID dose you now take. But be sure to consult with your physician before changing your dosage.

SAM-e: Better Cartilage and a Better Mood?

SAM-e is shorthand for s-adenosylmethionine, a chemical found naturally in all cells of the body. It plays a role in many biological reactions—in fact, it appears to regulate more than 30 different mechanisms—and deficiencies of SAM-e have been linked to several neurological disorders, including Parkinson's and Alzheimer's disease.

what the studies show

Chondroitin is somewhat more effective than glucosamine sulfate, according to an analysis of 15 clinical studies that was published in the March 15, 2000 issue of the *Journal of the American Medical Association*. The JAMA article concluded that glucosamine has a "moderately" positive effect in relieving pain and improving mobility, while chondroitin has a "large" positive effect.

In the late 1970s, Italian researchers studying SAM-e's effectiveness as an antidepressant noticed an unexpected side effect: some of their patients said the supplement helped relieve their arthritis pain. Today, SAM-e is one of the most popular dietary supplements, promoted not only for its ability to relieve depression but as a treatment for osteoarthritis as well. SAM-e does appear helpful for both problems, although there is more clinical evidence for efficacy against depression than for OA.

caution

SAM-e capsules and tablets may not always give you what you pay for. After analyzing eight SAM-e brands, the Good Housekeeping Institute reported that three of the brands contained less active ingredient than was listed on the label—and one of them (Nature's Vision) contained no SAM-e at all. Brands in which SAM-e content closely matched the label included Nature's Plus and Now.

How it works. Research hasn't yet shown how SAM-e works to relieve the pain of OA. Some evidence from laboratory and animal studies suggests that it may help rebuild damaged cartilage, but more study is needed to establish this effect. Preliminary studies suggest that SAM-e may actually have a disease-modifying effect on osteoarthritis.

BONING UP: Normally, the body manufactures all the SAM-e it needs from the amino acid methionine, which is found in common foods, including meats, soybeans, eggs, seeds, and lentils. However, a deficiency of methionine, choline, vitamin B_{12}, or folic acid can disrupt the body's ability to produce SAM-e.

As with glucosamine and chondroitin sulfate, SAM-e's usefulness as an arthritis treatment has been studied mainly in Europe. Some 10 clinical trials have indicated that SAM-e works as well as NSAIDs and better than placebos at relieving the pain of osteoarthritis. (There is no evidence that it can help against rheumatoid arthritis.)

Pricey Pain Relief

SAM-e is one of the most expensive of all dietary supplements. The price for taking enough of it to relieve arthritis pain may be prohibitively expensive for many people.

Studies showing SAM-e's effectiveness against arthritis pain have generally used doses of 1,200 mg per day. By contrast, a frequently recommended daily dose of SAM-e is only 400 mg. That would still cost you about $125 a month. . . which means that taking enough SAM-e to have an effect against arthritis pain could force you to spend $375 a month.

While 1,200 mg per day of SAM-e appeared to be well tolerated by patients in the clinical trials, it isn't recommended that anyone take that high a dose without first consulting their physician.

The bottom line. SAM-e may work as well as NSAIDs at relieving the pain of OA while causing fewer side effects. But its high cost means that SAM-e is not a treatment for everyone's pocketbook.

In one study in the mid-1980s, 734 patients with OA of the hip, knee, spine, or hand were assigned to take a daily dose of either 1,200 mg of SAM-e or 750 mg of the NSAID naproxen (Naprosyn). After one month, patients taking SAM-e reported pain relief that was similar to those taking naproxen and also experienced fewer side effects.

BONING UP: SAM-e often takes a few weeks to have a positive effect. It may be best to start with a minimum effective dose—400 to 600 mg per day.

Findings from this and other clinical trials were enough to persuade the Arthritis Foundation of SAM-e's usefulness. In 1999, the foundation issued a statement on SAM-e noting that its medical experts "feel that there is sufficient information to support the claim that SAM-e provides pain relief."

what the studies show

A double-blind study conducted in Germany showed that 36 patients with osteoarthritis who were treated with either SAM-e or ibuprofen derived the same degree of pain relief.

Collagen Supplements: Are They in Your Future?

Type II collagen is cartilage's major protein, providing cartilage with its tensile strength. Research suggests that type II collagen extracted from animals and taken orally can reduce the pain and inflammation of rheumatoid arthritis (perhaps by blunting the misguided immune attack responsible for the disease) while causing minimal side effects.

Promising studies. A study published in 1998 involving 60 RA patients found that those taking small doses of chicken collagen for three months experienced significant improvement in swollen and tender joints compared with patients taking a placebo. Similar clinical trials involving small numbers of patients were later carried out, with varying results.

Now, a company seeking FDA approval for its type II collagen product is sponsoring a major study involving nearly 800 RA patients. Results are expected soon and should go a long way toward showing whether type II collagen lives up to its promise.

You can already buy collagen II capsules in health-food stores, but don't assume that more is necessarily better: The clinical studies actually suggest that smaller doses may be more effective than larger ones.

The bottom line. Until results of the large-scale study are available, collagen II must be considered a promising but unproven treatment for RA. There is no evidence that it can help people with osteoarthritis. If you do try collagen II supplements, opt for a low daily dose of no more than 60 mg—the dose being used in the ongoing clinical study.

Cartilage Supplements: Don't Go There

At first glance it makes a lot of sense: Since osteoarthritis involves the loss of cartilage from the joints, restore the deficit by choosing one of the many cartilage supplements on the market, made from shark, cow, or other animals. But there are no studies to suggest that any cartilage product will help. True, glucosamine and chondroitin sulfate will be found in any cartilage product, but these two ingredients have been found useful only in purified form.

The bottom line. It's doubtful that cartilage supplements are of any use in treating arthritis.

Plant and Fish Oils: Modest Pain Relief

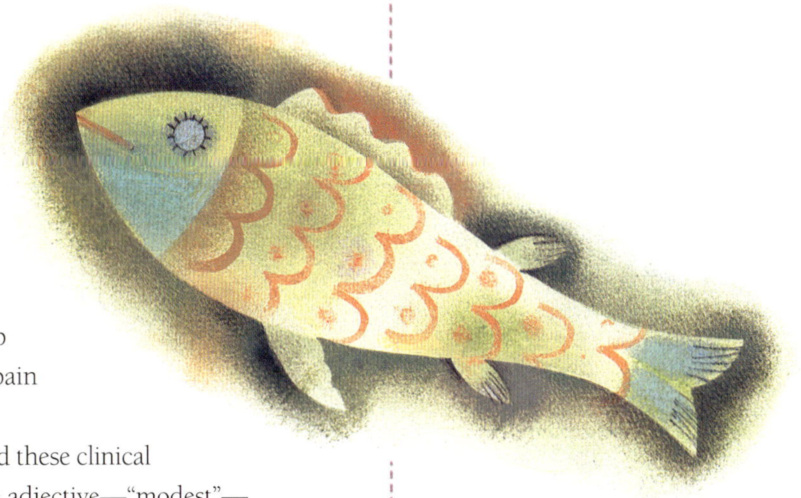

Oils obtained from fatty cold-water fish are rich in omega-3 fatty acids, which have the ability to decrease inflammation. By now some 20 clinical studies have shown that high daily doses of fish oil can help relieve the inflammation and pain of rheumatoid arthritis.

But experts who've evaluated these clinical studies invariably use the same adjective—"modest"—when describing the results. Furthermore, patients generally had to take fish oil for a long time—at least six months—before noticing improvement, and they had to take a lot of it: typically four to six grams a day, which can be expensive as well as unhealthy.

Taking fish-oil supplements in high doses can wreck your weight-loss efforts (they're basically fish fat, high in calories), increase your risk of bleeding problems by inhibiting clotting, and possibly raise your level of LDL cholesterol, the type associated with the clogging of arteries. Even more moderate doses can cause digestive problems, including upset stomach, diarrhea, and burping—and leave you smelling like a commercial fishing boat to boot.

Plant power. Oils pressed from the seeds of two weedy plants, evening primrose and borage, are rich in the fatty acid gamma linoleic acid (GLA). This fatty acid seems useful against the inflammation of RA, although it hasn't been studied as well as the omega-3s. But as with fish oil and its omega-3 cousins, patients must swallow a lot of evening primrose or borage oil to gain even modest improvement, and they run a risk for causing the same unpleasant side effects.

On the other hand, a mixture of oils extracted from avocados and soybeans—called piascledine—does help minimize the pain of hip and knee OA, according to two recent clinical studies

caution

Many evening primrose oil products reportedly are mixed with cheaper oils such as safflower or soy, which dilutes their effectiveness. Borage seed oils may contain low levels of potentially toxic chemicals called pyrrolizidine alkaloids; long term exposure to these chemicals can damage the liver and possibly cause liver cancer.

from France. In one of the studies, patients with severe OA of the knee or hip who took piascledine experienced less pain and disability after six months than patients taking a placebo. Improvements began after two months without any major side effects.

How it works. Although it is unclear how piascledine works, experts suggest that the oils may prompt chondrocytes (cartilage-making cells) to produce chemicals that help repair damaged cartilage. Piascledine was available only in Europe until recently but can now be purchased in the U.S. under the name, Avoca ASU.

The bottom line. RA patients must take fish oil, evening primrose oil, or borage seed oil for a long time for even modest improvement in symptoms. Little is known about whether any of these oils can help osteoarthritis patients. The possible side effects from these high doses may outweigh whatever benefits these oils offer. Piascledine may be helpful in treating OA.

The Antioxidant Advantage: C, E, and Beta Carotene

Growing evidence indicates that chemicals called free radicals may play a role in causing diseases associated with aging, including cataracts, heart disease, some types of cancer, and osteoarthritis. On the plus side, chemicals called antioxidants—particularly the vitamins C, E, and beta carotene that are found in many fruits and vegetables—can neutralize free radicals and prevent them from causing damage.

Damage control. Free radicals form constantly within the cells during normal metabolism, when the cells burn oxygen to create energy. The joints are among the places where free radicals are produced—and studies have shown that these chemicals can damage cartilage and may contribute to the damage that occurs in arthritic joints.

So could eating a diet rich in antioxidant vitamins—or taking them in the form of dietary supplements—help you ward off OA or perhaps ease its symptoms? Recent studies suggest that the answer is yes.

what the studies show

A German study found that taking 1,500 IU of vitamin E daily decreases pain and morning stiffness and improves grip strength in people with RA as well as the drug diclofenac does—without stomach upset.

BONING UP: Aspirin and other NSAIDs can alter your levels of iron, vitamin C, folic acid, and phosphorus and decrease your body's ability to absorb these important nutrients.

The famous Framingham Heart Study, in which researchers have followed the residents of Framingham, Massachusetts, for nearly 50 years, has shed light on other health problems besides heart disease. In one study, the Framingham researchers looked for evidence of OA of the knee in 640 people who were evaluated during two exams spaced about 10 years apart. The subjects also filled out a questionnaire asking about their dietary intake.

The study found that people who took in more than 180 mg of vitamin C per day were only one-third as likely as people consuming half that amount to have their OA worsen over 10

did you know

Bioflavonoids may help strengthen cartilage and possibly lessen its chances of becoming inflamed. Bioflavonoids are found in virtually all plant foods—fruits, vegetables, legumes, grains, and nuts.

Alternative Therapies: How to Break It to Your Doctor

Don't keep it a secret: Inform your physician about the alternative treatments you use. Herbs and other supplements can cause side effects and dangerous drug interactions, possibly entailing costly tests or treatments if your doctor doesn't know you've been using them.

Mum's the word. Surveys show that 40 to 60 percent of people who use alternative therapies don't disclose that fact to their physicians, presumably for fear of ridicule or criticism. But you probably needn't worry, since physicians today are much more accepting of alternative therapies than just a few years ago.

A *Consumer Reports* survey found that when people felt comfortable enough to inform their doctors about their alternative choices, a majority of the doctors (55 percent) expressed approval. Some 40 percent took a neutral stance, and only 5 percent disapproved.

caution

People on prescription blood-thinning drugs (anticoagulants) or aspirin should consult their doctor before using vitamin E (which also thins the blood).

years—a benefit due mainly to reduced cartilage loss. In addition, people with OA who consumed vitamin C in moderate or high amounts were much less likely to develop knee pain.

Findings for vitamin E and beta carotene were also positive, but not quite as impressive as for vitamin C. People consuming the highest amounts of beta carotene had half the risk of seeing their OA worsen compared with people consuming the least amount. And for vitamin E, the benefits were more modest and limited to men: those who consumed the most vitamin E were significantly less likely to have their OA worsen compared with men in the lowest category.

The bottom line. It's premature to recommend antioxidant supplements for preventing or treating arthritis—the evidence for benefit comes from too few studies. But for people concerned that they don't eat the recommended five to nine daily servings of fruits and vegetables, supplementing your diet with vitamin C (the antioxidant that seems most helpful against arthritis) may be a good idea.

what the studies show

Antioxidants may also help against rheumatoid arthritis. Two small studies have found that people with a low intake of vitamins C, E, and beta carotene were more likely to develop RA than people with higher intakes.

Vitamin D: Beef Up Your Bones and Cartilage

Vitamin D is synonymous with bones, since it helps the body absorb calcium, the key ingredient in bone. But since bones in a joint are literally joined to their cartilage, vitamin D could influence osteoarthritis as well.

How it works. Researchers believe that a bone's "integrity"—its ability to withstand weight-bearing activities and other stresses—may affect whether OA worsens or not. So for people with OA who also have "soft" bones—perhaps because of inadequate vitamin D intake—OA may be a more serious problem. Vitamin D also affects cartilage directly, by stimulating the cells that produce cartilage to make more of it.

Knowing all this, the Framingham researchers decided to investigate whether dietary vitamin D might influence OA, and they carried out their study the same basic way as their antioxidant study mentioned above.

Get 'Em from Foods First

In general, it is best to get as much of the vitamins and minerals you need from your diet, not from a supplement. Foods contain phytochemicals and other potentially beneficial compounds not found in pills that may help in your battle plan against arthritis.

If your diet would make a nutritionist wince, then add a daily multivitamin/multimineral supplement to your regimen to supply the missing nutrients. In the case of vitamin E, it might be difficult to reach the often-recommended 200 to 400 IU from diet or a multivitamin. In this case, you probably want to consider taking a single supplement of that vitamin daily.

BONING UP: Fortified milk contains about 100 IU of added vitamin D per cup. The milk used to make yogurt, cheese, and other dairy products usually isn't fortified, however, so these foods contain only trace amounts of vitamin D.

In addition to vitamin D from food, people synthesize their own vitamin D when their skin is exposed to sunlight—which is why it is also called the sunshine vitamin. So the researchers assessed not only the vitamin D in people's diets but also—to get a more complete idea of the vitamin's presence—measured the level of D in their blood.

Persuasive proof. Vitamin D was found to have an important influence on OA. People who consumed little vitamin D and had low levels in their serum were three times more likely to experience a worsening of their knee OA compared with people who had high intakes and high serum levels. In addition, low serum levels of the vitamin were associated with loss of cartilage in the knee.

The bottom line. If you have OA, make sure that you're consuming the Recommended Dietary Allowance of vitamin D

When D Becomes Toxic

Since vitamin D is a fat-soluble vitamin, it's not excreted readily and can easily build up to toxic levels in your tissues. Too much vitamin D can cause calcium deposits in the body, resulting in serious damage to the kidneys and cardiovascular system.

Play it safe by avoiding single-nutrient vitamin D supplements. If you drink a couple of glasses of vitamin D-fortified milk per day, taking D supplements could actually spill your intake into the danger zone.

each day, which is 400 International Units (IU). Based on the results of the Framingham study, that should be enough to keep your bones and cartilage healthy. You can further bolster your vitamin D levels by getting more sun exposure or simply by taking a multivitamin containing 400 IU of vitamin D.

Herbal Solutions: Don't Be Green About Their Claims

Herbal products have been used for thousands of years to treat virtually every human ailment, including arthritis. But despite the dozens of herbs purported to treat arthritis, patients in the U.S. have largely steered clear of them—at least when it comes to treating their condition.

For example, in its recent survey of alternative-therapy use, *Consumer Reports* found that only a small percentage of arthritis patients who used alternative therapies opted for herbs—and the ones they used (echinacea, garlic, and ginkgo biloba) are not generally used for treating the condition.

Boning Up: **Boswellin is a gum derived from a tree native to India. In animal studies, it has been shown to inhibit inflammation and prevent the loss of glycosaminoglycans, which are important components of cartilage.**

what the studies show

Green tea contains compounds called polyphenols, which may help relieve RA inflammation. In one study, green tea extract was found to cut the rate of arthritis in animals taking it. Green tea is available in capsules, or drink it the old-fashioned way. Don't add milk to your tea, though—it may block the effects of the beneficial polyphenols.

The bottom line. If you are interested in trying herbal remedies for arthritis, be aware that evidence for their effectiveness is almost entirely anecdotal. Herbs that may show some benefit against arthritis and seem reasonably safe include angelica (also known as wild celery), boneset (feverwort), ginger, and boswellin.

Even if an impassioned friend tells you about his or her miraculous experience with one herb or another, resist the seduction: Check with your doctor first or do your homework online or in a library. Natural is not synonymous with nontoxic, especially when you are also taking prescription drugs—which can interact dangerously with herbs.

what the studies show

In one study, people with RA showed decreases in pain, stiffness, and joint tenderness and swelling, and inflammation, and improvement in grip strength after four months of taking a combination of four plant extracts: boswellin, ginger, curcumin (the active component in turmeric), and withania somnifera (also known as ashwagandha).

Other Treatments: What's Hype, What's Not

Ever since Neanderthal man woke up with stiff, achy joints, man has been looking for an antidote—standard remedies, alternative approaches, home remedies, anything. Some are reasonable and safe; others don't have a scientific leg to stand on. Here are some that fall into both categories.

Antibiotics: For RA Patients Only

Antibiotics are useful for treating Lyme arthritis and other types of arthritis that are caused by bacterial infections. Antibiotics also show promise in easing the inflammation of rheumatoid arthritis—but not for the reasons you might think.

Researchers have long suspected that viruses or other microbes play a role in triggering RA. Yet decades of intensive searching have turned up little evidence to support the notion. As a result, the beneficial effects of minocycline—the antibiotic that seems most useful against RA—apparently have nothing to do with killing bacteria or any other organisms.

How they work. When antibiotics are administered, many of them can affect human cells—in ways that have nothing to do with their action against microbes. Research on minocycline (a

MSM: The Sulfur Connection

The dietary supplement MSM (methyl sulfonyl methane) has been promoted for treating arthritis and many other health problems. This sulfur compound is found in a number of foods including milk, fish, grains, and fresh fruits and vegetables. Sulfur is an important element in chemicals that make up cartilage—and MSM is destroyed when food is processed—leading proponents to claim (without any scientific support, mind you) that MSM is the answer to arthritis problems.

An unproved remedy. Sold as a dietary supplement in powder, pill, and lotion form, MSM is classified as an unproved remedy by the Arthritis Foundation, despite the praises sung by actor James Coburn, who touts it as a magical solution to chronic rheumatoid arthritis.

member of the tetracycline family of antibiotics) suggests that it muffles the immune response that causes RA while at the same time suppressing cells responsible for the destructive enzymes that inflame the joints of RA patients.

The bottom line. Three well-regarded clinical trials suggest that minocycline may offer a genuine benefit in treating RA, especially in the early stages of the disease. If you have RA and aren't satisfied with your current therapies, you may want to talk with your physician about trying minocycline.

Copper Bracelets: Jewelry, Not Therapy

Copper's use as a therapeutic agent was noted in an Egyptian papyrus prepared in 1550 B.C.—and wearing copper bracelets to combat arthritis pain may date back almost that far. The copper in bracelets is indeed soluble in human perspiration. But there is no good evidence that copper eases the inflammation or pain of arthritis. Actually, copper levels in the blood of rheumatoid arthritis patients are *higher* than normal—casting further doubt on copper's usefulness.

The bottom line. By all means wear a copper bracelet if you like its appearance, but don't expect it to ease your arthritis.

DMSO: Risky Business

DMSO (dimethyl sulfoxide) is used mainly as an industrial solvent. A cleaning fluid similar to turpentine, DMSO has been touted as a treatment for numerous health problems, including arthritis, cancer, mental illness, stroke, multiple sclerosis, and varicose veins. The FDA has approved DMSO for treating interstitial cystitis (an uncommon bladder disease), but not for any other medical purposes.

Side effects. The chemical has been shown to cause damage to the lens of the eye in animal studies and can be potentially toxic to the liver in humans. The most common side effects are skin rashes, headache, nausea, and diarrhea.

The bottom line. DMSO has not been well studied as an arthritis treatment—and the available evidence provides little assurance that the solvent is effective or safe.

Magnet Therapy: Proving Its Mettle?

Unless you've been living in a cave for the past couple of years, you've probably been hearing about "the healing power of magnets." They've recently been promoted for their ability to ease the pain of arthritis and carpal tunnel syndrome, heal injuries, improve circulation, and provide relief from asthma and other medical problems.

But don't throw away your heating pad or ibuprofen. Magnets may be attracting a lot of buyers, but they haven't yet proven their mettle.

Magnetic appeal. Medical magnets can be bought in sporting good stores and pro shops, through the mail, and over the Internet. You can purchase them individually, as thin strips containing numerous magnets, and in many other forms, including magnetic headbands (for headaches), mattress pads (for arthritic joints and backache), and shoe insoles (for sore feet).

How they work. One theory holds that magnets improve blood flow, delivering extra oxygen and nutrients to the area while reducing toxins. The best evidence that magnets offer medical benefits arose from a small, highly publicized study on pain relief carried out at Baylor College of Medicine in Houston and published in 1997. This study involved 50 people suffering from the pain of postpolio syndrome; 29 of them had magnets placed over their painful areas for 45 minutes, while the other

did you know

Magnet therapy dates back to the ancient Greeks. Hippocrates reportedly used the magnetic rock lodestone to treat sterility.

21 received comparable treatment from sham magnets that looked exactly like the real ones.

The findings: 76 percent of the people treated with the real magnets reported a decrease in pain, while only 19 percent of those treated with sham magnets noticed any improvement. That's a significant difference—but each patient was treated only once, and the study failed to note how long the pain relief lasted.

BONING UP: **There are clear differences in the different brands of magnets on the market. If you try one particular brand and it fails to relieve your pain, don't give up. Try at least two others.**

The bottom line. So far, no published studies have shown that magnets can ease the pain of osteoarthritis or any other type of arthritis. On the other hand, magnets are relatively inexpensive and—unless you have an electronic pacemaker—apparently safe to use. So if you're drawn to trying magnets for arthritis pain, there's no harm in giving them a try.

Mind Over Matter: Short-Circuiting Stress

It is arthritis' version of a vicious circle: That flare of knee pain you woke up with this morning is making you angry and anxious. You were going to visit a friend on the other side of town and now, thanks to those sharp stabs, you think you have to cancel it. What may not know is that your stressful emotions could very well be turning up the volume on your pain.

Just Relax: Techniques to Tone Down the Tension

The stress response. When pain is a chronic problem, stress can become chronic, too—and it can make a bad case of arthritis even worse. How? Stress can lower your pain threshold and can tighten muscles around the joints, literally squeezing them and limiting their range of motion.

But, as it turns out, you don't have to put up with the painful fallout of stress. You can, as you have with everything else affecting your condition, take charge. There are proven self-help techniques that can cut the legs out from under tense emotions. In fact, clinical studies have shown that arthritis patients who regularly use such techniques can reduce their pain and improve their mobility. Next time your pain gets the best of your emotions, try one of these relaxing strategies:

Biofeedback. This technique vividly illustrates mind over matter, training the mind so that it can control physiological functions such as heart rate and blood pressure. A machine using electrodes attached to the patient's skin records subtle physical processes, such as pulse rate, heart rate, or even muscular tension. These processes are measured on the biofeedback machine as electrical signals or sounds. With practice, you can learn how to control these internal functions—by changing your thought patterns, for example, or visualizing a pleasant scene. Eventually, as you learn what mental technique produces the desired change, you'll be able to produce those physical changes on your own—without the equipment.

BONING UP: Stress reduction may be especially important for people with rheumatoid arthritis, since studies suggest that stress may worsen symptoms of the disease by disrupting immune function.

Studies show that biofeedback can relieve stress and pain associated with fibromyalgia, rheumatoid arthritis, and chronic pain associated with osteoarthritis. Learning to relieve your symptoms this way may take just a few biofeedback sessions or as many as a couple of dozen.

Visualization. This technique channels the power of the imagination to create changes in the body—namely, relieving stress and easing the pain and other symptoms of arthritis. As you

what the studies show

In a study published in 1996, researchers looked at 19 studies comparing NSAID treatment alone for arthritis with treatment that included NSAIDs and mind-body techniques. Compared with NSAID treatment alone, mind-body treatments provided an additional 20 percent improvement in symptoms for OA patients and an extra 20 to 40 percent boost for RA patients. Mind-body therapies were especially helpful in improving the functional ability of RA patients and decreasing their number of tender joints.

recognize yourself getting tense, conjure up a peaceful setting—lying on a tropical beach, for example, or looking out on a sea of sunflowers on a summer day. Alternatively, you can visualize yourself doing some desired activity—working in the garden, for example—and doing it effortlessly and without pain. Or you can tackle your pain head-on, imagining that the pain is red and hot. Gradually, visualize the color changing to a cool blue as it fades. To enhance the results of visualization, choose a quiet, dimly lit room and ask that your family not disturb you for awhile.

Guided imagery. This is essentially "visualization" plus—namely, through the aid of a mental health professional or other practitioner who "guides" you through the mental exercises. The therapist will first put you through exercises to help you relax and then facilitate visualizations that may help yield relief for your symptoms.

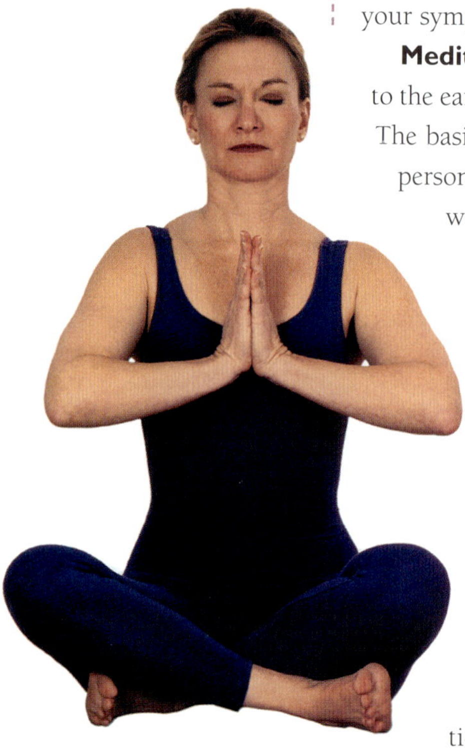

Meditation. This approach dates back thousands of years to the earliest religions and includes many different techniques. The basic intent of all meditation techniques is to influence a person's consciousness by redirecting his attention in some way—focusing on your breathing, for example, or a single word, thought, or object to rid your mind of all other thoughts and feelings.

Meditation helps diminish arthritis symptoms by diminishing the stress that worsens them. The term "relaxation response," in fact, grew out of the meditation research of Harvard physician Herbert Benson, who showed that a simple meditation technique (just sitting in a quiet place and focusing on any phrase or sound) can induce physiological changes, such as lowered heart rate and blood pressure, in practically anyone.

Not surprisingly, the more you practice meditation, the better you will get at it—and the more benefits you will achieve. Try meditating at least three or four times a week.

Beyond Relaxation: Help for the Depressed

Not everyone will be rescued by mind-body therapies. For some people, arthritis can simply be too much to cope with. The stress from their pain and disability creates a level of anxiety, depression, or other emotional problems that only a mental-health professional can allay. It's understandable how a chronic disease like arthritis can overwhelm you emotionally. Managing it can dominate your life: taking medications, going to doctor's appointments, going online to find out about the latest research, trying new treatments that are not helping your pain.

BONING UP: **Support groups, either face-to-face or online, are an effective way to deal with emotional problems caused by arthritis. According to Dr. Ronald C. Kessler at Harvard, self-help groups have become one of the most important treatments for dealing with emotional problems in the U.S.**

Making the call. If you feel overwhelmed by your arthritis—and friends and family haven't made a dent in your funk—there are options. You can call a professional counselor who might be able to lift you out of your gloom. Professional counselors serve at all levels of schools and universities, mental health agencies, and hospitals. Common ways to locate a counselor include referral from your physician or calling the National Board for Certified Counselors (336-547-0607).

There are many different types of mental-health professionals and many different types of therapies to choose from. One therapy—cognitive behavioral therapy—may be particularly suited for painful conditions such as arthritis. In fact, the National Institutes of Health has endorsed the use of this therapy for easing the pain of both OA and RA.

How it works. The aim of cognitive behavioral therapy is to get patients to focus on their negative thoughts, and to recognize the link between their negative way of thinking and the stress or depression they're feeling. Once patients realize that their negative attitude is not only distorted but contributes to their emotional turmoil, they may take a more positive approach that helps lift depression and stress.

what the studies show

- A 1998 survey of arthritis patients found that 29 percent were extremely depressed but that few of them received any intervention for their depression. And studies have found that rates of depression among patients with rheumatoid arthritis are seven times higher than the rate for the general population.

- A study published in 1999 in the *Journal of the American Medical Association* found that people with mild to moderately severe rheumatoid arthritis could significantly ease their symptoms by writing about stressful experiences.

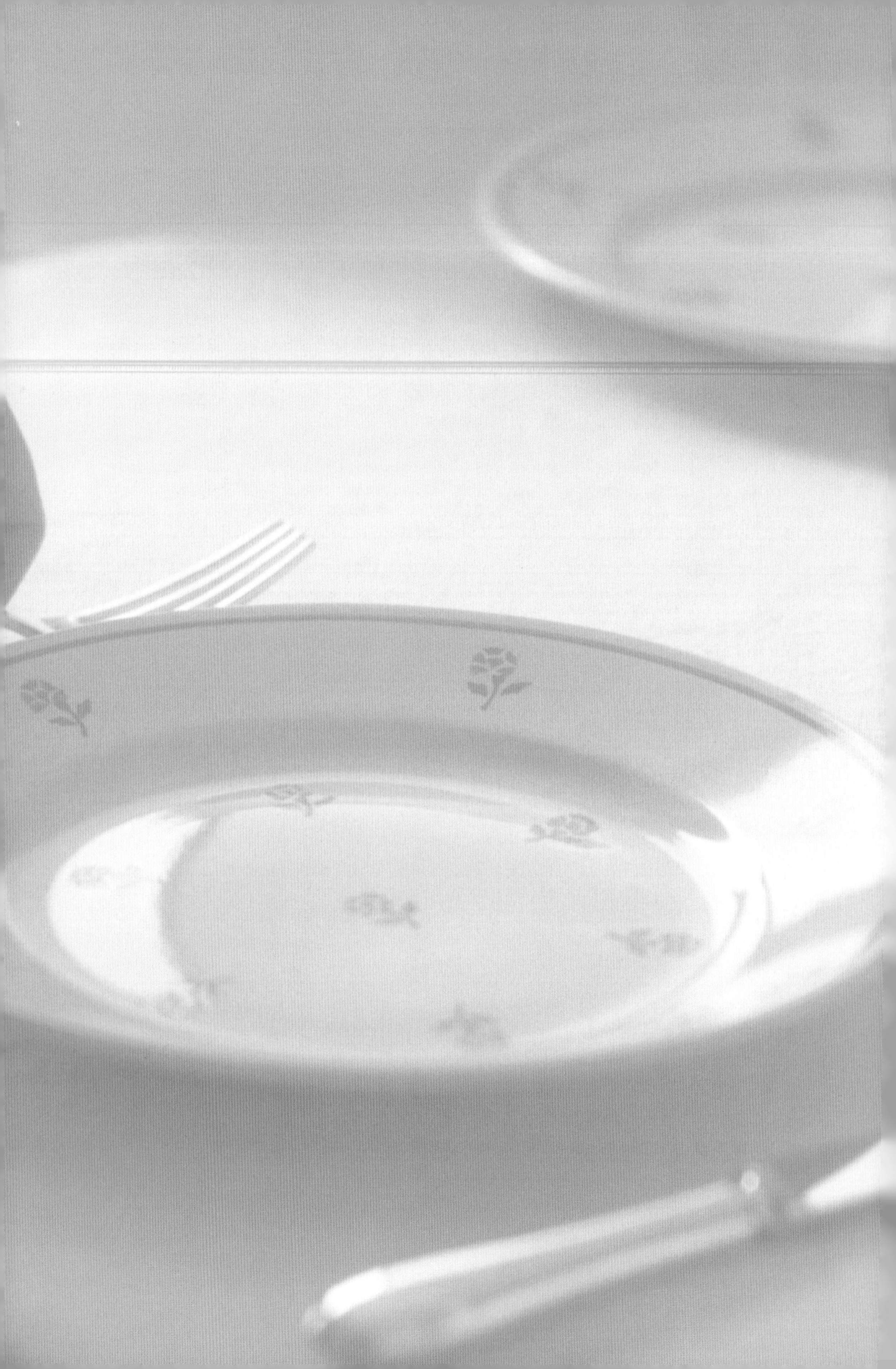

7

Eating to Beat Arthritis

Perhaps the best medicine for your arthritis isn't something you can buy in the drugstore, but something you can buy in the grocery store. The right foods have helped many patients improve their condition.

KEY CONCEPT

Taking charge of your diet enables you to take charge of your disease three times a day. This is especially true for osteoarthritis sufferers who are overweight.

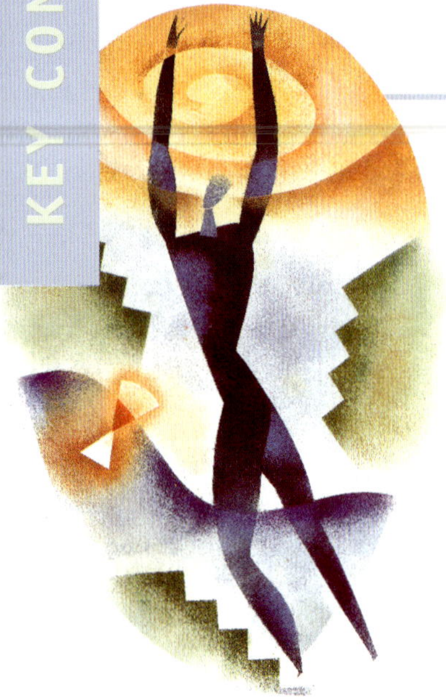

Weighty Issues

There really is no upside to carrying around extra pounds: It increases your risk of developing a host of serious conditions—heart disease, some cancers, diabetes, and—yes—osteoarthritis. What's more, if you are already diagnosed with arthritis and are also overweight, you will suffer the consequences more than your slimmer counterpart: The extra pounds can cause further damage to your joints and worsen pain and stiffness.

Not surprisingly, losing weight can protect your joints and significantly ease your symptoms. But there's much more to "diet" than just calories. Recent studies show that eating foods rich in certain vitamins and other nutrients can slow down the progression of osteoarthritis and ward off its symptoms. Some of these nutrients seem to help protect the joints from damage—something that not even drugs can do.

Overweight and OA

Piling on extra pounds is now recognized as a major cause of osteoarthritis. And judging by recent surveys showing that more than half of all Americans are overweight, it may be the most important cause of all. In particular, overweight can cause OA of the weight-bearing joints—the knees and, to a lesser extent, the hips. But it is also associated with a greater risk of OA in other joints as well, including the back, ankles, big toes, and hands.

The pressure of pounds. When you think about it, obesity's role in causing OA—or in aggravating symptoms in people who already have the disease—makes all too much sense. The protective cartilage that covers the ends of the bones in a joint is just a few millimeters thick. Years of carrying around spare pounds puts extra pressure on the knees and other weight-bearing joints, grinding down cartilage to the point that bone rubs against bone and giving rise to the pain and stiffness of OA. In people who already have OA, being overweight can speed up cartilage loss and cause the disease to worsen.

Studies have documented the overweight-arthritis link. They've followed groups of people over several years, keeping close tabs on their weight and whether they developed OA. One study involved more than 1,000 women age 45 to 64 who lived in London; 58 out of the 67 women with OA in one knee returned for a follow-up X ray two years later. Of the 32 clearly overweight women, 15—or nearly half—had by then developed OA in their other knee as well; but only one of the 10 normal-weight women had gone on to develop OA in her other knee.

Losing It: The Upside of Slimming Down

The good news is that overweight people who lose weight can prevent OA of the knee from occurring. This was first demonstrated in a study published in 1992—the first ever to show that OA was potentially preventable. And the weight loss didn't need to be dramatic: By losing just 11 pounds over a 10-year period, the study found, an overweight woman could reduce her risk for developing OA of the knee by 50 percent.

The vicious cycle. When it comes to OA, being overweight is notorious for pushing patients down that long and slippery slope paved with increasingly more severe symptoms. Once people develop arthritis, there are often reasons—many of them totally understandable—why patients continue to put on weight or can't take it off. Arthritis sufferers frequently become depressed, which can lead to overeating that adds even more pounds. In addition, someone with stiff, sore joints tends to

did you know

It's normal for body weight to fluctuate a few ounces during the course of a single day, mostly due to changes in water content. Those who weigh themselves daily (or worse yet, several times a day) may become obsessed with the numbers on the scale, panicked when there is a slight gain, or overly confident when there is a loss. Weigh in, at most, once a week.

prefer the couch to the track, leading to more weight gain and even worse pain and disability.

Unfortunately, the health impact of too many pounds goes beyond arthritis. Being overweight can increase your risk for developing many other health problems as well—high blood pressure, adult-onset diabetes, heart disease, and several types of cancer, including prostate cancer and colorectal cancer.

did you know

Eliminating obesity in the U.S. would lower the incidence of OA of the knee by 25 to 50 percent and would reduce the incidence of OA of the hip by 25 percent or more.

Are You Packing Pounds?

For most of us, figuring out if we're overweight is painfully easy: a glance in the mirror will usually suffice, and then there are the pants that are too snug or the collars that no longer button. Half of our total body fat is wedged between the muscles and the skin, so we can usually sense when there is too much of it. But more scientific methods are also available, including the height-weight chart below.

The chart is intended for use by both men and women and has some wide ranges for each category. Note that people who

Do You Weigh Too Much?

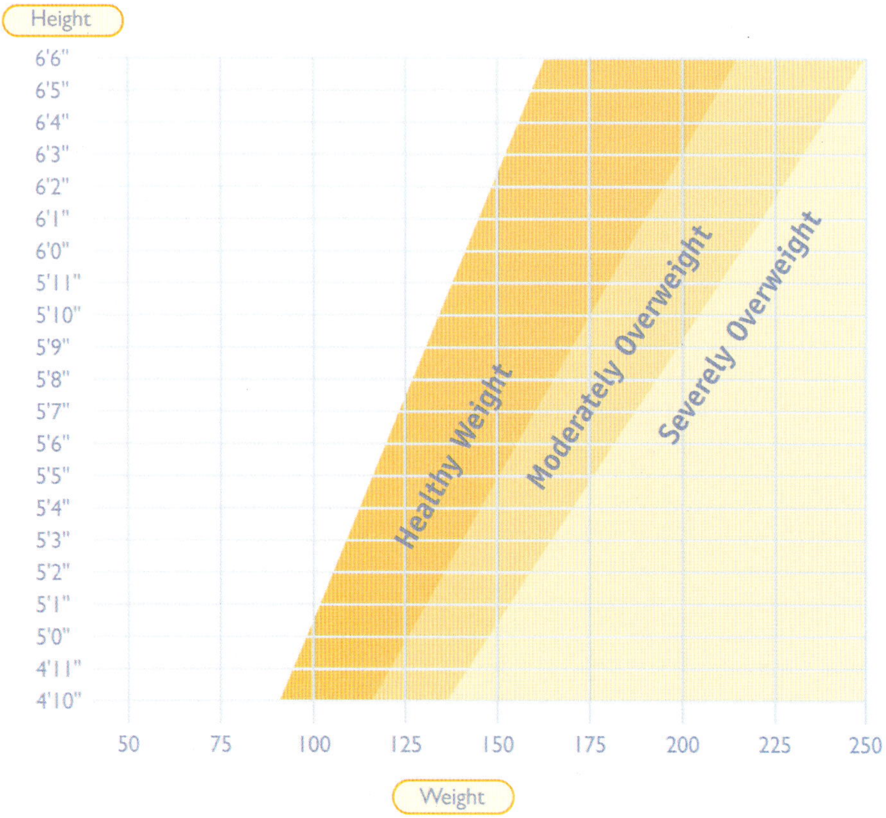

Weight Loss Winners: Principles to Lose By

Many diets fail because they involve dramatic changes that only the most resolute can stick with. The better and more enduring approach is reshaping your eating habits a little at a time. Here are some winning tips:

- Make changes for yourself, not to please others. You want to lose weight, keep fit, and reduce your osteoarthritis symptoms. You can't do it just because your spouse or your best friend has nagged you into it.
- Record everything you eat to pinpoint your weaknesses. Do it for a week, including the weekend as well.
- Focus on making wise food choices rather than resisting temptation. Very few win the willpower game.
- Don't throw out yummy foods. Instead, satisfy your urges with appealing alternatives such as baked potato chips instead of the deep-fried varieties.
- Don't let yourself get too hungry. Skipping one meal leads to overeating at the next. Passing on breakfast can leave you hungry all day.
- Get at least some exercise everyday. Keeping your body in motion raises your basal metabolic rate so you burn calories faster than before, even when resting.

are the same height can differ by more than 25 pounds and still fit into the "healthy weight" range—mainly because two people the same height can have widely differing amounts of "heavy" muscle and bone. (Men, with their greater muscle and bone mass, usually weigh more than women of the same height.)

You shouldn't assume that you're home free just because you're within the upper limit of "healthy." Even small weight gains within the range of healthy weights may increase your risks for health problems. But if you're muscular, have a large frame and are generally in good health, then your weight is probably satisfactory.

The Great Pyramid: Eat to Lose

Healthy eating involves much more than just playing bean counter and adding up long lists of calories you consume. The idea is not only to lose weight if you need to but also to eat the right kinds of foods: those that are low in fat and high in beneficial nutrients such as fiber and vitamins.

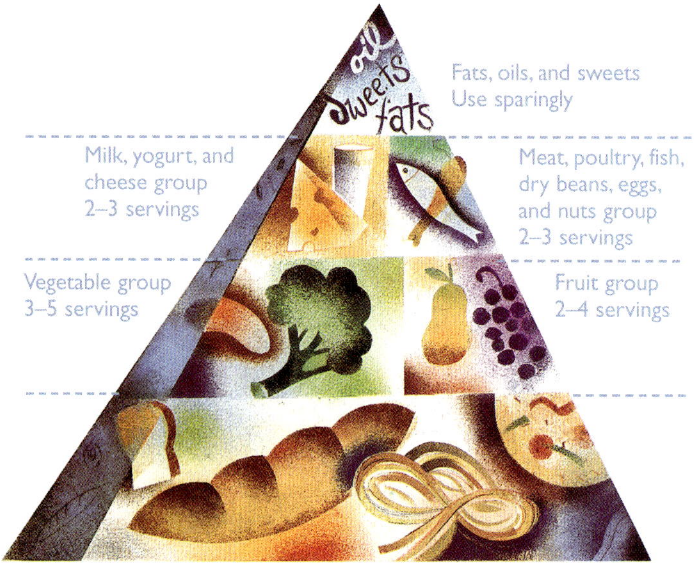

Optimally, this approach to eating will be not only effective but also practical—an eating strategy that you can stick with over the long haul without feeling deprived or bored.

One eating approach does meet those requirements, but it doesn't receive the hype of the Zone Diet, the Atkins Diet, or the other highly touted fad diets that publishers trot out with regularity. It's known as the Food Guide Pyramid (left) and was developed by the U.S. Department of Agriculture.

Losing it for good. The food pyramid is intended to guide you in choosing the types of foods to eat each day. It has two crucial advantages over its flashier (and flash-in-the-pan) competitors: You'll have a better chance of sticking with it for life, and nutrition experts regard it as the healthiest eating strategy yet devised.

Sticking with the food pyramid diet can help people with OA lose weight if necessary and then maintain the healthy weight they've achieved. Equally important, the pyramid can help you ward off or reduce your risk for developing cancer, heart disease, diabetes, hypertension, and other health problems associated with being overweight. The diet accomplishes these aims by emphasizing the three factors that are key to healthy eating: balance, variety, and moderation.

A Guide—Not a Diet

Some 50 million Americans are dieting at any one time—and you may well be among them. If so, your hopes of slimming down will almost inevitably end in disappointment.

Extensive research and surveys of dieters themselves all show that any reducing diet or commercial diet program can produce significant weight loss—and even produce it rapidly. But the ultimate goal is to keep that weight off, and the vast majority of dieters are not able to do that. Almost inevitably, they promptly regain all the weight they lose on diets.

Focus on food. The great virtue of the Food Guide Pyramid is that it's not a diet but a healthful approach to eating. It doesn't focus on calories but emphasizes the food groups that are best for long-term good health: grains, fruits, and vegetables. These foods are high in health-promoting vitamins, minerals, and other nutrients and low in saturated fat, cholesterol, and calories.

BONING UP: It's best to get your nutrients from whole food rather than supplements. Foods contain a host of other beneficial substances that can be critical to minimizing your symptoms.

Not surprisingly, pursuing the pyramid's recommendations will almost inevitably mean reducing your calorie intake and losing weight in the process—and having an excellent chance of maintaining that weight loss.

Climbing the Pyramid: A Stairway to Dieting Heaven

If you include the number of servings of food recommended in the Food Guide Pyramid, you'll have little appetite left for the chips and Snack Wells. Still, the pyramid does provide you with enough latitude to keep your diet interesting. The key is to make the right choices within each food group.

did you know

- More than half the calories that people take in are burned up in basal metabolism—the energy we expend to stay alive.
- Many people aren't aware that they need fewer calories as they get older. Not only does their metabolism slow down but they also tend to become less active. So maintaining a healthy weight as you get older may require trimming your calorie intake.
- The Japanese government suggests eating at least 30 different foods a day. By eating many different kinds of foods, it's almost certain that you will get a wide variety of nutrients. And most people can't overdo it on any one kind of food when they have 29 other kinds to fit into their diets.

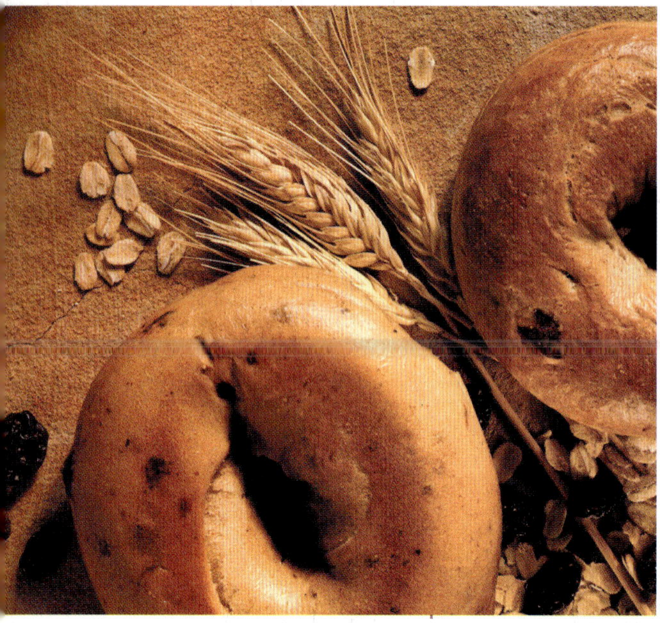

Start—and stay—with grains

The lowest level of the food pyramid consists of grains—bread, cereal, rice, and pasta. Grains are quite literally the pyramid's foundation and are the foundation of a healthy diet as well. The message is to go to the grains more than any other food.

Grains—especially whole-grain varieties in which the fiber and vitamins and minerals haven't been removed—provide complex carbohydrates (starches) that supply the body with energy. Contrary to what you may think or have heard, these starches are not fattening—provided you omit the butter and other high-fat toppings like full-fat cheese or sour cream, or sugary confections. In addition, pasta and other grains have the virtue of leaving you feeling satisfied.

BONING UP: Eat mostly whole grains that are high in fiber. Because most fiber leaves the body undigested, your body doesn't absorb the calories it contains.

Serving information: You should try to give grains the starring role in your diet and aim for 6–11 servings per day, most of them from whole-grain varieties. A single serving consists of either 1 slice of bread, 1 ounce of cereal, ½ bagel or English muffin, 1 small roll, biscuit, or muffin, 3 to 4 small or 2 large crackers, or ½ cup cooked rice or pasta.

Produce power

The next tier of the pyramid is composed of fruits and vegetables. Both are nature's attempt at diet food—low in fat and calories and rich in flavor, fiber, phytochemicals, and antioxidant vitamins that are especially important for anyone suffering with osteoarthritis.

Luckily, it's not as hard as you might think to make fruits and vegetables a bigger part of your diet—and to improve your joints and your overall health in the process. You just need some point-

what the studies show

Studies have shown that fiber-rich foods are a natural appetite suppressant. Because they take up more room in your stomach than other foods, you feel fuller faster. Fiber is slower to digest, so it keeps hunger at bay longer. And most fiber-rich foods simply take more time to chew (think granola vs. doughnut), so your brain has more time to register that you've had enough—before you've had too much.

Antioxidants for Arthritis

Findings from the landmark Framingham study indicate that the antioxidant vitamins C, E, and beta carotene help to prevent the progression of osteoarthritis. Antioxidants help to neutralize free radicals, chemicals continually formed within cells during normal metabolism that can damage cartilage and possibly cause inflammation as well.

So what are the best sources of antioxidants? Fruits and vegetables, of course. Here is a Cliffs Notes approach to maximizing your daily antioxidant intake. Eat...

- Red grapes rather than green or white varieties
- Red and yellow onions instead of white
- Cabbage, cauliflower, and broccoli raw or lightly cooked
- Garlic raw and crushed
- Fresh and frozen vegetables rather than canned ones
- Microwaved vegetables instead of boiled and steamed ones
- The deepest, darkest green leafy vegetables
- Pink grapefruit instead of white grapefruit
- Whole fruits rather than juices
- Fresh and frozen juices instead of canned ones
- The deepest orange carrots, sweet potatoes, and pumpkins

ers in stealth nutrition—sneaking in produce with your three squares. By following these suggestions, you can boost your intake of fruits and vegetables right away:

- Begin your day with six ounces of 100 percent fruit juice (three-fourths of a cup) and you've taken care of one serving.
- Garnish your cereal with sliced bananas, berries, raisins, or other fruit. You need only one-fourth cup of dried fruit, half a cup of berries, or one medium piece of banana or other fruit to make a full serving.

did you know

The antioxidant impact of fruits and vegetables extends far beyond vitamins C, E, and beta carotene. Produce also contains hundreds and perhaps thousands of different phytochemicals (substances found only in plants). Many of them appear to function as antioxidants, and only a small fraction of them have been identified.

BONING UP: Want to eat more fruit? Put it out where you can see it. People are more likely to eat fruit that's in a bowl on a counter than in a refrigerator—and much more likely than if it's in the dining room.

- Make your omelet using plenty of vegetables—onions, peppers, tomatoes, or any other that appeals to you. Half a cup of chopped vegetables provides you with one serving.
- Prepare your lunchtime salad using chicory, romaine, or spinach. (Avoid iceberg lettuce, the least nutritious of all vegetable greens.) One cup of raw, leafy vegetables gives you one serving.
- Add tomatoes, sliced peppers, shredded carrots, or bean sprouts when making sandwiches.

Where the Vitamins Live

Now that you know what anitoxidant vitamins can help your arthritis, where are you going to get them? Here is a guide to what foods contain which nutrients:

Beta carotene: Yellow-orange fruits and vegetables such as apricots, sweet potatoes, pumpkin, carrots, cantaloupe, mangoes, papaya, peaches, and winter squash, as well as dark green leafy vegetables such as broccoli, spinach, collard greens, parsley, and other leafy greens.

Vitamin C: Cantaloupe, grapefruit, papaya, kiwi, oranges, mangoes, raspberries, pineapples, bananas, strawberries, tomatoes, and fresh vegetables such as Brussels sprouts, collard greens, cabbage, asparagus, broccoli, potatoes, and red peppers.

Vitamin E: Sunflower and safflower oils, sunflower seeds, wheat germ, nuts, avocados, peaches, whole-grain breads and cereals, spinach, broccoli, asparagus, dried prunes, and peanut butter.

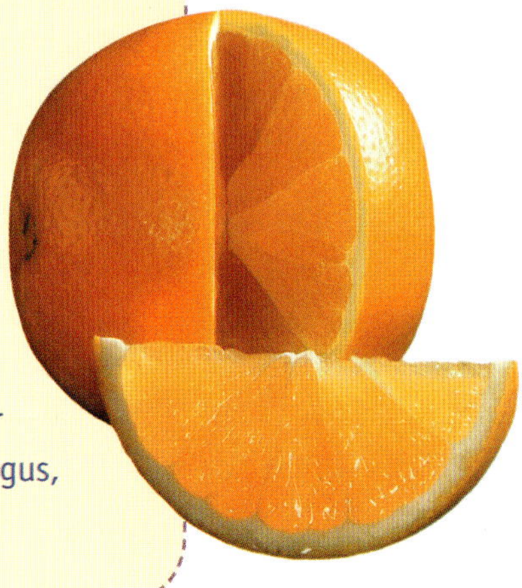

- When it's time for a healthy snack, don't settle for sticks of celery or carrots. Expand your snack menu to encompass raw broccoli, cauliflower, green beans, summer squash, and red and green peppers.
- Take along raw vegetables as a side dish when you're brown-bagging your lunch.
- Drink fruit or vegetable juices rather than taking a coffee or tea break. Buy a case of small boxes or cans of juice that are easy to carry with you.
- When you prepare pasta for dinner, remember that a half cup of tomato sauce qualifies as a serving of cooked vegetable.
- Prepare several fruit desserts each week, such as poached pears, or that blast from the past, Jell-O with pieces of fruit.
- Frozen yogurt becomes tastier and healthier if you add berries or sliced apples, bananas, peaches, or plums.

Serving information: Strive for 3-5 servings of vegetables and 2-4 servings of fruits daily. A single serving of vegetables is ½ cup cooked or raw vegetables, 1 cup leafy raw vegetables, ½ cup cooked legumes, ¾ cup vegetable juice. A single serving of fruit is 1 medium apple, banana, or orange, ½ grapefruit, 1 melon wedge, ¾ cup juice, ½ cup berries, ½ cup diced, cooked, or canned fruit, ¼ cup dried fruit.

Got milk? Or cheese? Or fish?

The third tier of the food pyramid includes the dairy group—milk, yogurt, and cheese—and the meat, poultry, fish, dry beans, eggs, and nuts group. By now, you have probably noticed that the further up the pyramid you proceed, the fewer the number of daily servings that are called for. That's by design, of course. The lower-calorie, more nutrient-rich foods reside at the bottom.

Dairy products provide most of the calcium in our diets. In addition, they are our main source of vitamin D, which—although not an antioxidant—is crucially important when it comes to osteoarthritis.

what the studies show

Researchers at the University of North Carolina at Chapel Hill recently measured levels of 11 antioxidant phytochemicals in the blood of 200 people with OA of the knee and 200 people who did not have the problem. Having elevated blood levels of several phytochemicals—beta cryptoxanthine, lutein, and lycopene—was associated with a 30 to 40 percent reduced risk for developing OA. These phytochemicals are found in leafy green and brightly colored vegetables. Tomatoes, for example, contain high levels of lycopene.

caution

To be on the safe side, avoid single-nutrient vitamin D supplements. If you happen to be consuming a couple of glasses of vitamin D-fortified milk a day, taking D supplements could actually tip your intake into the danger zone.

Serving information: Shoot for 2 to 3 servings per day (4 for pregnant/lactating teenagers). A single serving is 1 cup of milk or yogurt, 2 ounces of processed cheese food, or 1½ ounces of cheese.

BONING UP: Always opt for low-fat or nonfat dairy products. Full-fat milk and cheese are high in fat and calories—the prime ingredients for weight gain. Lower-fat varieties provide the same beneficial nutrients as their full-fat brethren.

The power of protein. Meat, poultry, fish, dry beans, eggs, and nuts are your best sources of protein and also supply you with B vitamins, iron, and zinc. Obviously, the lower-fat choices in this category are beans or fish, but there are wise ways to cut fat from meat.

Trimming the fat before cooking, removing the skin before eating, and choosing leaner cuts of red meat at the grocery store can make the difference between a high-fat and slimmer meal. When choosing beef, look for leaner "choice" cuts rather than "prime" cuts. With poultry, light meat is lower in fat than dark meat—by about 50 percent

Serving information: Shoot for 2 to 3 servings per day. A single serving consists of 2-3 ounces of cooked, lean meat (about the size of a deck of cards), poultry, or fish, or ½ cup cooked dried beans (1 egg or 2 tablespoons of peanut butter count as one ounce of meat).

Sweet somethings

At the pyramid's apex sits the fat, oils, and sweets group—along with the notation to "use sparingly." These calorie-rich foods offer little in the way of nutrition, which is why they're known as "empty calorie foods." Examples include fat-filled foods such as salad dressings, butter, and margarine, and sugar-rich foods such as candies, cakes, and soft drinks. With their copious calories and especially their high fat content, these foods can pose a major stumbling block to your weight-loss efforts.

what the studies show

A 1996 study found that vitamin D has an important influence on osteoarthritis. Researchers found that people who consumed less than the U.S. Recomended Daily Allowance of vitamin D (400 International Units) were about three times more likely to experience a worsening of their knee OA compared with people who exceeded the RDA for vitamin D. Based on this study, meeting or slightly exceeding the vitamin D RDA of 400 IU daily should be sufficient for keeping your bones and cartilage healthy.

Ferreting Out the Fat

Meat, full-fat dairy products, nuts, oils, and desserts are responsible for most of the fat in people's diets. If you are overweight, cutting back on the fat in these foods is job one. Gram for gram, fat contains more than twice as many calories as carbohydrates or protein (9 calories in a gram of fat vs. 4 in a gram of carbohydrate or protein).

Adding insult to injury, researchers now know that not all calories are the same: Calories from fat are the worst for weight-conscious consumers, since they are more efficiently stored as fat in the body than are calories from carbohydrates or protein. On top of the extra weight it causes, a diet high in fat—especially the saturated fat found in animal products—harms the body in other ways, such as raising blood cholesterol levels and increasing the likelihood of developing certain cancers.

Over the past 25 years—thanks in part to cutting back on red meat and emphasizing leaner foods such as chicken, turkey, and fish—Americans have modestly pared the percentage of total calories they derive from fat: from an average of 41 percent down to 36 percent. But we can do better. The government recommends restricting the percentage of their calories from fat to 30 percent; many experts believe that fat consumption should be much lower, with no more than 15 or 20 percent of calories from fat.

did you know

Consider using fruit juices or fat-free chicken or beef broth instead of butter or oils when sauteeing vegetables.

A Calorie Calculator

Here's a shorthand way to tally up the calories you take in when consuming servings from the Food Guide Pyramid:

Food Group	One serving provides about
Grains	80 calories
Vegetables	25 calories
Fruit	60-80 calories
Meat, poultry, fish, dry beans, eggs & nuts	150-250 calories
Milk, yogurt, and cheese	150-200 calories

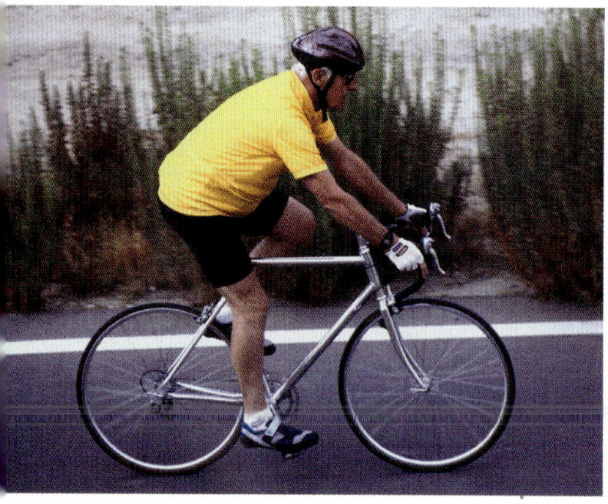

BONING UP: Regular exercise can be extremely effective in weight control. In fact, study after study shows that dieting alone can help people lose weight—but that exercise is needed to keep it off.

What to do? Fortunately, by making some minor substitutions among the foods you buy, you can significantly reduce the amount of fat—and the percentage of calories from fat—in your diet. The following table illustrates some major differences in fat among foods that otherwise are quite similar. To single out one example: Pretzels and potato chips are both salty snacks, but there is a dramatic difference: one ounce of potato chips contains 11 times more total fat than one ounce of pretzel twists.

Fats in Foods

Food		Total fat in grams	Calories	% of cal from fat
Tuna	Chunk light in water, 3 oz., undrained	1.0	89	10
	Chunk light in vegetable oil, 3 oz., undrained	17.6	254	62
Chicken	Roasted light meat, no skin, 3.5 oz	4.5	171	24
	Fried, battered, light meat, with skin, 3.5 oz.	15.3	274	50
Meat	Sirloin steak, lean only, broiled, 3 oz.	7.7	180	39
	Sirloin steak, lean & fat, broiled, 3 oz.	15.7	240	59
Milk	Skim milk, 1 cup	0.4	86	4
	Whole milk, 1 cup	8.1	150	49
Ice Cream	Vanilla-flavored premium ice milk, 4 fl. oz.	2.9	100	26
	Vanilla ice cream, 4 fl. oz.	17.9	260	62
Snacks	Pretzel twists, 1 oz.	0.9	110	7
	Potato chips, 1 oz.	11.7	160	66

Reading the Fat Print

Knowing your way around the nutritional analysis labels found on virtually all food packaging can save you calories and fat. Here are the facts behind fats:

- Fat-free: Less than 1/2 gram of fat per serving (remember, a package often consists of more than one serving)
- Low-fat: 3 grams of fat or fewer per serving
- Reduced fat: At least 25 percent or less fat than its full-fat product
- Light or lite: 1/3 less calories or 50 percent less fat

Example: If a label reads "light doughnuts" (meaning 50 percent less fat than regular doughnuts), that doesn't mean you have the green light to eat it. You should know that regular doughnuts are very high in fat, so that a light doughnut probably still has a lot (in fact, 10 grams down from 20).

Make Changes Slowly

Changing something as basic as what you eat—tofu instead of steak, say—can be difficult indeed. You're most likely to succeed over the long term if you proceed gradually. Here are some tips for making modest changes that, over time, can really add up:

- If you use cream in your coffee, switch to whole milk for a few weeks, then to reduced fat (2 percent) milk, then to low-fat (1 percent) and finally to nonfat (skim milk).
- Eat more slowly. By doing so, you'll find that you feel satisfied with smaller portions.
- Move meat, chicken, and fish from center stage on your plate and make vegetables the largest serving.
- Cut recipe amounts of meat in half; use only lean meats (look for round or loin on the package), and fill in the lost bulk with shredded vegetables, legumes, pasta, grains, or other low-fat items.

- Opt for variety. When you go to the supermarket, buy a fruit or vegetable that you've never tried before.
- When you leave for work or for a day's outing, bring your food along with you to avoid buying fat-filled fast food.

Watch Those Portions!

Nutrition experts all seem to agree: Americans have a greatly exaggerated idea of what size a serving should be. Restaurants in particular deserve blame for implanting the idea of supersizing in the minds of consumers.

BONING UP: One sure way to sabotage a diet, experts agree, is to rule out certain foods entirely. Rather than consider any food forbidden, you should instead eat small portions of it fairly regularly. For example, instead of denying yourself your weekly whole deep-dish pizza, plan to have just one or two slices instead.

In fact, the clear trend in the U.S. has been toward consuming larger food portions (see *Size Does Matter*, right), especially of foods rich in fat and sugar. The result? Not surprisingly, an unbalanced diet. At the same time, the collective waistline has been expanding as a nation, suggesting an increasing need to control portion sizes if we are to win the battle of the bulge.

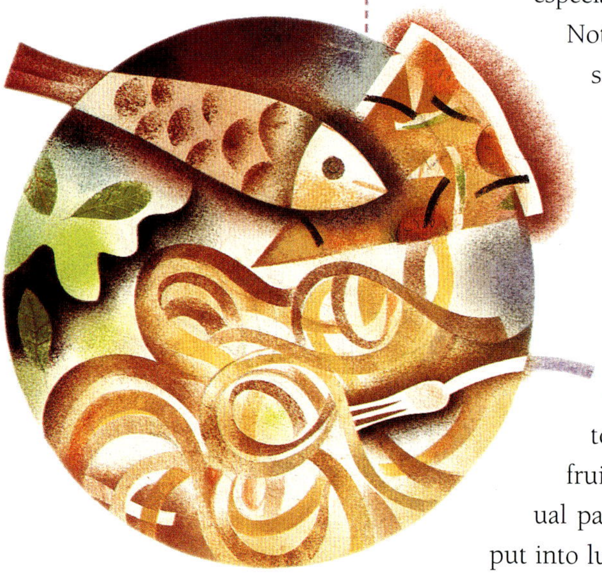

This distorted notion of serving size not only piles on the calories but also gives many people the mistaken idea that consuming the recommended five to nine servings of fruit and vegetables is a feat akin to scaling Everest. But actually, one serving of fruit is just a half cup—the size of the individual packs of applesauce or fruit salad that moms put into lunch boxes for their first-graders.

Size Does Matter

This chart underscores the larger portion sizes that have become part of our culture:

Food	Food Guide Pyramid	Typical Portion 1977	Colossal Portion 2000
Cola	—	10 oz. bottle, 120 cal.	40-60 oz. fountain, 580 cal.
French fries	10, 160 cal.	About 30, 475 cal.	About 50, 790 cal.
Hamburger	2-3 oz. meat, 240 cal.	3-4 oz. meat, 330 cal.	6-8 oz. meat, 650 cal.
Steak	2-3 oz., 170 cal.	8-12 oz., 690 cal.	16-22 oz., 1,260 cal.
Pasta	1/2 cup, 100 cal.	1 cup, 200 cal.	2-3 cups, 600 cal.
Baked potato	3-4 oz., 110 cal.	5-7 oz, 180 cal.	1 pound, 420 cal.
Candy bar	—	1 1/2 oz., 220 cal.	3-4 oz., 580 cal.
Popcorn	—	1 1/2 cups, 80 cal.	8-16 cup tub, 880 cal.

From the book *Nutrition: Concepts and Controversies*

Diet Therapy for Arthritis: Does It Work?

The notion that some foods can make arthritis worse while others might ease its symptoms is both intriguing and controversial. Until recently, most experts were skeptical about diet therapy's role in arthritis and considered it the nutritional equivalent of snake oil.

But studies over the past few years have shown that some dietary interventions may be of some use, particularly for patients with inflammatory forms of arthritis such as rheumatoid arthritis. Here's a rundown of the main ways that diet has been used to treat arthritis—and what the evidence shows.

Can You Scale the Pyramid?

Ideally, you'll want a diet that approximates the recommendations of the Food Guide Pyramid. Keeping a food diary will give you feedback on whether your diet provides the proper number of servings of each food type and whether you're getting a sufficient variety of foods.

For each meal, fill in your number of servings of each food group. Then, at the end of the day, tally up the totals for each group. Don't get discouraged. Breaking well-entrenched habits can't be done overnight.

Breakfast	Number of Servings
Bread	________
Vegetable	________
Fruit	________
Dairy	________
Meat	________
Lunch	
Bread	________
Vegetable	________
Fruit	________
Dairy	________
Meat	________
Dinner	
Bread	________
Vegetable	________
Fruit	________
Dairy	________
Meat	________

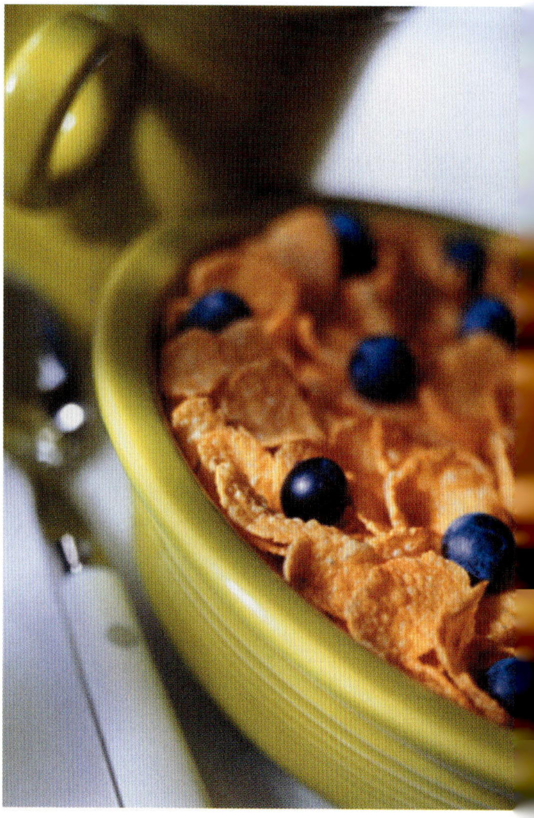

Totals for the Day

Bread group servings	________
Vegetable group servings	________
Fruit group servings	________
Dairy group servings	________
Meat group servings	________

Avoidance Diets

These are based on the idea that certain foods are the aggressors when it comes to arthritis. By subtracting the offending foods from your diet, proponents claim, people with arthritis will experience significant improvements in their symptoms.

The anti-nightshade diet. Probably the best known of the avoidance diets, it's based on the idea that members of the "nightshade" family of foods—tomatoes, potatoes, eggplant, and peppers—contain chemicals that not only promote inflammation but also increase pain and interfere with the repair of damaged joints.

The "nightshade theory" was proposed by a horticulturist who knew that tomatoes and other nightshades were once considered poisonous—and noticed that they seemed to worsen his arthritis. He carried out an uncontrolled study in which more than 5,000 arthritis patients were asked to avoid nightshade foods for seven years; nearly three-quarters of the patients said their pain and disability gradually improved with the diet.

The bottom line. The nightshade-free diet has never been studied in a scientifically rigorous way, though some rheumatologists have reported that a few of their patients improved after nightshades were removed from their diets. It can't hurt to try the diet (provided you don't make radical dietary changes that could interfere with nutrition), but don't expect much from it.

The Dong diet. Named for the physician who devised it for his own arthritis—Collin Dong—the Dong diet is patterned after one that many Chinese have followed for centuries. The Dong approach imposes much broader food restrictions than the anti-nightshade diet. Arthritis patients are urged to eat vegetables (except for tomatoes) but to eliminate red meat, fruit, dairy foods, herbs, alcohol, soft drinks, and additives and preservatives.

In a study published in 1983, some arthritis patients were placed on the Dong diet while others consumed a diet allowing for a variety of foods. No significant differences were noted, with about half the people in each group reporting that they felt better.

The bottom line. No scientific evidence supports the Dong diet, which could actually harm people who have arthritis: The diet excludes fruit, which provides antioxidants and other nutrients that are important for the health of joints; and it bans dairy products, the main dietary source of the calcium and vitamin D needed to maintain bones and assist in cartilage formation.

did you know

Nightshades come from the plant genus *Solanum* and include more than 1,700 herbs, shrubs, and trees, including eggplant, bell peppers, potatoes, and tomatoes. Although there are many claims that removing nightshades from the diet will cure arthritis, no scientific proof has yet been offered.

Eliminate the Negative?

If you suspect that a particular food such as tomatoes makes your arthritis worse, it can't hurt to eliminate that food from your diet and then wait for a couple of weeks to see if you feel better. A more scientifically rigorous—but more drastic—approach is dietary elimination therapy, which should be done only under a doctor's supervision.

This therapy begins with a food "exclusion" phase, designed to clear the system of all possible food culprits. The exclusion phase may require a total water fast lasting for a week or a less extreme, more nourishing diet consisting perhaps of fish, pears, carrots, water, and other foods considered safe to eat. If your symptoms do disappear during the exclusion phase, foods are then carefully reintroduced one at a time to see which ones are actually causing the problem.

Anti-Allergic Diets: Have They Caused a Reaction?

Many arthritis patients are convinced that some foods—particularly milk products, corn, and cereals—do more than just aggravate their arthritis, but can actually trigger symptoms in a matter of minutes, much as people with asthma may start coughing after inhaling pollen or other substances to which they're allergic.

Some people do have genuine food allergies, in which a food protein prompts the immune system to produce antibodies against that protein, which is known as an antigen. Antibody combines with antigen to form antigen-antibody "complexes." Proponents of the allergy-arthritis notion contend that these antigen-antibody complexes could conceivably irritate the joints or even attack the joints' synovial lining.

Experts now believe that food sensitivities such as allergies may be involved in some cases of rheumatoid and other types of inflammatory arthritis. But the actual proportion of patients affected appears to be quite small—perhaps five percent or fewer. Consider the results of one carefully done study that involved 159 patients with rheumatoid arthritis, 52 of whom claimed that food aggravated their symptoms. Actual testing of all the patients failed to detect a single case of food intolerance.

Diets That Put Out the Fire?

Inflammation is the body's response to tissue damage or to overuse of a diseased joint. Researchers have found that fatty acids may alter for the better the inflammation response in certain types of arthritis, as can certain chemicals found in teas.

Fishing for Relief

Studies of Greenland Eskimos led to interest in the anti-arthritic properties of fish. Although they lived mainly on fatty fish, these Eskimos were found to have a remarkably low level of heart disease—and of rheumatoid arthritis as well. The beneficial effects of these cold-water fish were attributed to their fat, specifically the omega-3 fatty acids that are plentiful in fish oil.

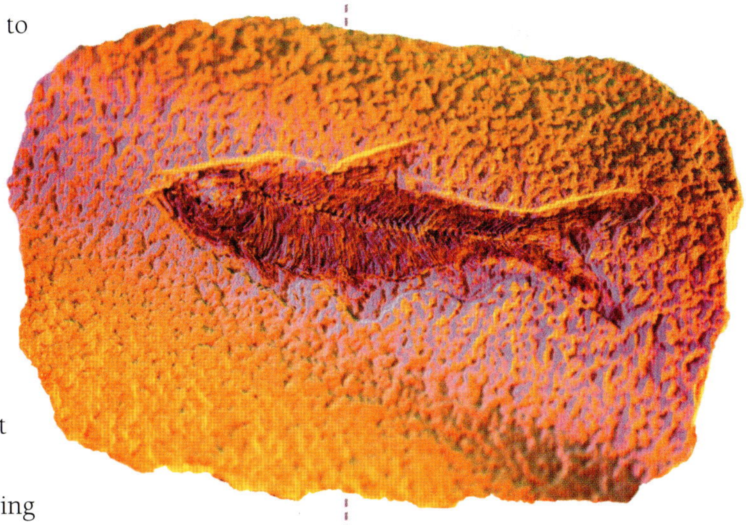

Researchers now know that eating fish can help reduce inflammation in several ways. For example, a diet high in fish changes the lipids that make up cell membranes in the body, and this change reduces the level of inflammatory chemicals called cytokines.

Several studies have shown fish-oil supplements may offer modest benefits in easing symptoms in patients with rheumatoid arthritis, for whom inflammation is a key problem. But it isn't known yet whether fish-oil supplements will benefit people with osteoarthritis—which typically doesn't involve inflammation.

Even if fish or fish-oil supplements don't help to ease your arthritis symptoms, consuming more fish makes a lot of sense. Studies show that people who eat fish regularly can gain some important health benefits.

Fat Content of Selected Seafood

Food (3 oz.)	Omega-3 fatty acids (g)	Saturated fat (g)	Total fat (g)	Calories
Atlantic salmon	1.9	1.1	6.9	155
Herring	1.8	2.2	9.8	172
Whitefish	1.6	1.0	6.4	146
Bluefin tuna	1.3	1.4	5.3	156
Sardines, canned, in oil	1.3	1.3	9.7	177
Mackerel	1.1	3.6	15.2	223
Rainbow trout	1.0	1.4	5.0	128

BONING UP: Eicosapentaenoic acid (EPA), best known of the omega-3 fatty acids, is found in marine plants and fish. EPA is actually made by algae, plankton, and seaweed, which are then eaten by certain fish.

A major study of American men found that those consuming the most fish were about 40 percent less likely to die from a heart attack or clot-caused (thrombotic) stroke over a six- to eight-year period than men who consumed the least amount of fish. In addition, researchers have found that omega-3 fatty acids—the kind plentiful in fatty fish—are important nutrients for vision, for nerve and immune function, and possibly for protection against several types of cancer.

The bottom line. All fish contain some omega-3 fatty acids. But to maximize your intake, choose oily cold-water fish such as salmon, tuna, and mackerel (see the table above). Eating cold-water fish two or three times a week should help your overall health and could be of some help for your arthritis.

caution

Too much fish or fish oil can interfere with your blood's ability to clot. Excessive intake of fish oil can lead to overdoses of vitamins A and D (especially if you're getting A and D in your vitamin supplements), which can be toxic.

Sip Your Arthritis Symptoms Away?

If you have arthritis or simply want to improve your general health, you should take a cue from the English and the Asians and have a spot of tea. Researchers have long known that tea is rich in flavonoids, a class of phytochemicals known for its antioxidant abilities. Some studies have shown that regular tea drinkers are up to 50 percent less likely to develop certain types of cancer compared with nontea drinkers, while other studies have found that regular tea drinkers have a lower risk of stroke and heart disease. And as noted earlier in this chapter, evidence suggests that diets rich in antioxidants can help keep osteoarthritis from worsening.

The green light to green tea. Both black and green teas are good sources of flavonoids. But now there is reason to believe that green tea may be particularly useful against rheumatoid arthritis, thanks to a different class of phytochemicals known as polyphenols, present in abundant amounts in green tea.

Researchers at Case Western Reserve University School of Medicine in Cleveland extracted the polyphenols from green tea leaves and added them to drinking water fed to young mice. An identical group of mice received water without polyphenols. Later—after all the mice were injected with a chemical that usually triggers a disease resembling RA—the mice who had consumed the polyphenols were much less likely to develop RA, and the cases that did occur were milder. Fewer than half the polyphenol-drinking mice even developed RA, compared with 94 percent of those drinking plain water.

The bottom line. Try drinking three or four cups of green tea daily without milk to see if it reduces inflammation. Note: Green tea does contain caffeine (about 40 mg a cup), so to compensate, you may want to cut back on other sources of caffeine such as coffee.

did you know

Letting green tea steep more than five minutes can cause the beneficial substances to lose their potency. Use one teaspoon of green tea leaves per cup of very hot (not boiling) water.

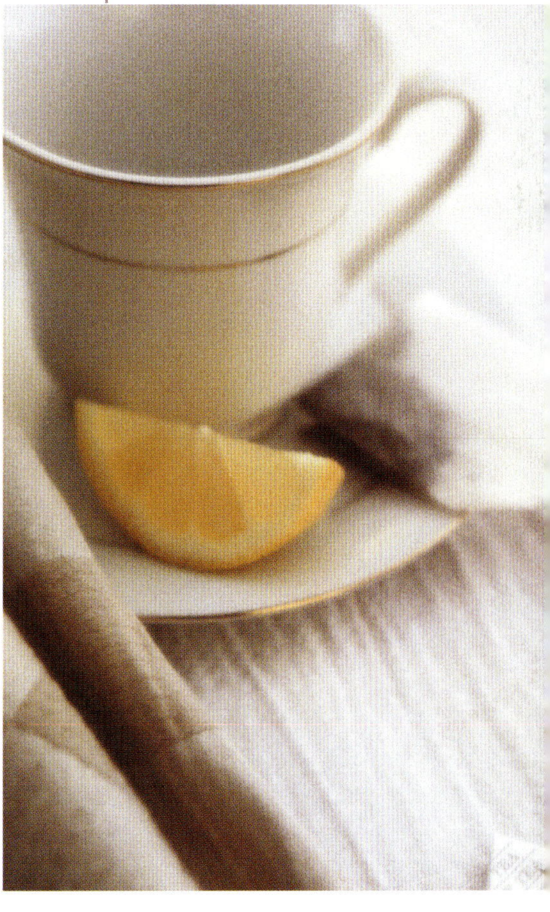

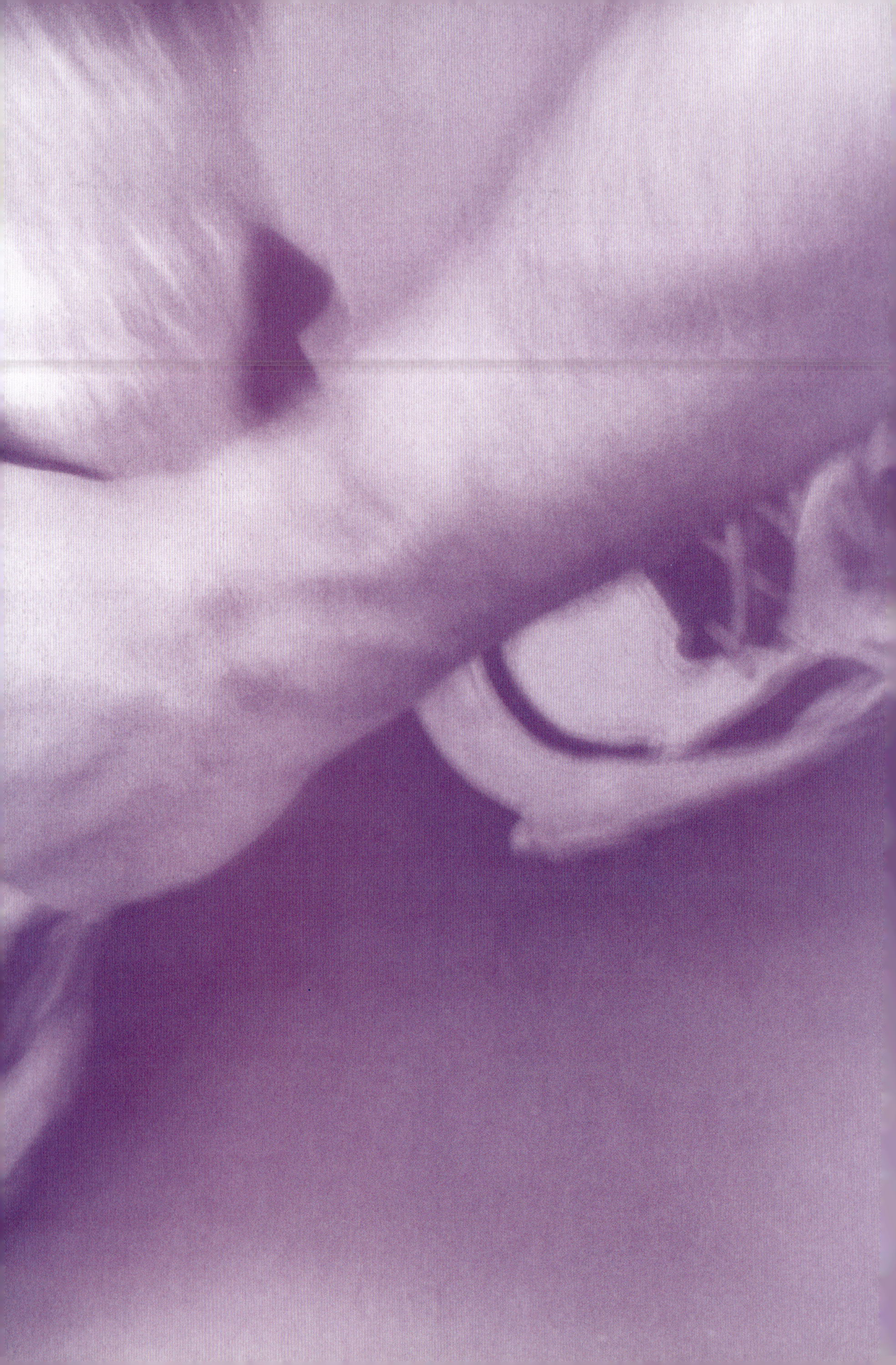

8 Get Moving

The human body is built to move. That might seem painfully contradictory to an arthritis patient with a knee joint that feels like hardening cement. But exercise is indeed medicine in motion: It can help prevent osteoarthritis, and it can certainly help those already hobbled with the condition.

KEY CONCEPT

Exercise is one of the pillars of the take-charge movement. It is not only vital for weight loss—a boon for anyone with arthritis of the knee or hip—but also essential to the health of your joints.

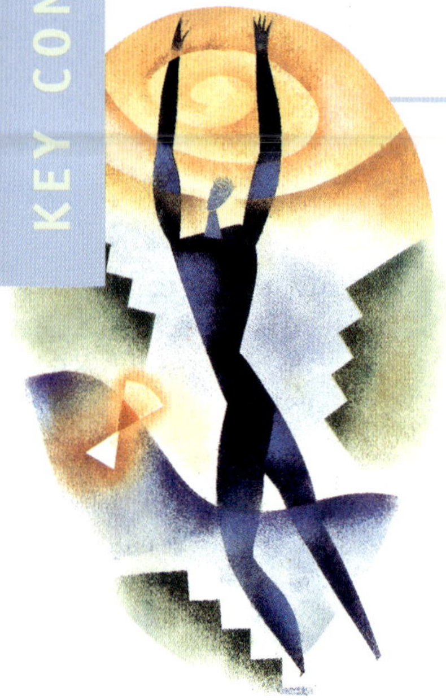

The Call of the Couch Potato

Exercising an arthritic joint seems counterintuitive: When a joint has that achy, breaky feeling, any person in his or her right mind wouldn't think that swimming, cycling, or walking would make it better. But it does. Inactivity leads to the wasting away of muscle, which can increase the strain on joints that causes even more pain.

Until a few years ago, doctors perpetuated their patients' predilections toward inactivity by advising them to stay off their feet. They assumed that osteoarthritis was an inevitable part of aging and that exercise just made things worse by speeding up cartilage destruction. As for patients with rheumatoid arthritis, doctors believed that joint-jolting exercise would do nothing but trigger inflammation and flare-ups.

The healing power of movement. Wrong. Science, fortunately, has had the last word on the subject, proving that exercise is good medicine for arthritis sufferers. Study after study has shown that moderate activity does not damage joints or worsen arthritis pain. In fact, regular exercise is one of the best therapies for relieving joint pain and also improves many other health problems common to arthritis patients.

A Smorgasbord of Benefits

Arthritis can cast a pall not just on a person's joints, but also on her health profile: Studies show that many people with arthritis have poor overall health, especially when it comes to risk factors for heart disease. Compared with "nonarthritic" people the same age, arthritis sufferers tend to be much heavier and have higher blood pressure, lower levels of HDL cholesterol (the "good" form that prevents heart disease), and higher blood sugar levels (indicating possible diabetes). The reason? Inactivity—which was recently declared a major heart-disease risk factor.

BONING UP: **Strong, well-toned muscles, tendons, and ligaments can bear the brunt of the force that crashes into joints as we move. In fact, the majority of the load that the joints bear can be transferred to these supporting structures, taking some of the load off the cartilage.**

did you know

One of every eight people over age 65 experiences limitations of activity due to arthritis.

Small Moves, Big Gains

Scientific evidence shows that doing moderate exercise regularly will net you the following laundry list of benefits:

- Reduced risk of death from all causes
- Reduced risk for developing heart disease
- Reduced risk for hypertension (and lowered blood pressure in people who are already hypertensive)
- Help in weight loss and weight management
- Reduced risk for several types of cancer, including colon, prostate, and possibly breast cancer
- Reduced risk of stroke
- Improved blood glucose control in people with type 2 (adult-onset) diabetes and less risk of diabetes-related complications
- Reduced anxiety and depression
- Improved quality of sleep

Exercise offers numerous health benefits to people no matter what their age or their physical condition, but it can be especially valuable for people with arthritis. Regular activity can relieve pain and stiffness as effectively as NSAIDs and other drugs—while offering two crucial additional advantages:

- Drugs—especially the pain-relieving NSAIDs—can cause serious and potentially fatal side effects, while exercise rarely causes significant problems.
- Drugs and exercise can both relieve symptoms, but exercise does something that no drug can do: modify the course of arthritis by making joints healthier—stopping osteoarthritis from worsening and perhaps even preventing the disease from occurring.

Besides relieving pain and stiffness, the right combination of exercises can help strengthen and stabilize arthritic joints and prevent them from becoming deformed. Equally important, exercise can reduce the mental stress that can amplify physical pain. Need further motivation to get moving? Staying active can lower your risk for heart disease, diabetes, hypertension, and several types of cancer; provide relief from insomnia and depression; and improve immunity and one's sense of well-being.

did you know

When muscles are immobilized—through complete bed rest, for example—they can lose 3 percent of their strength each day.

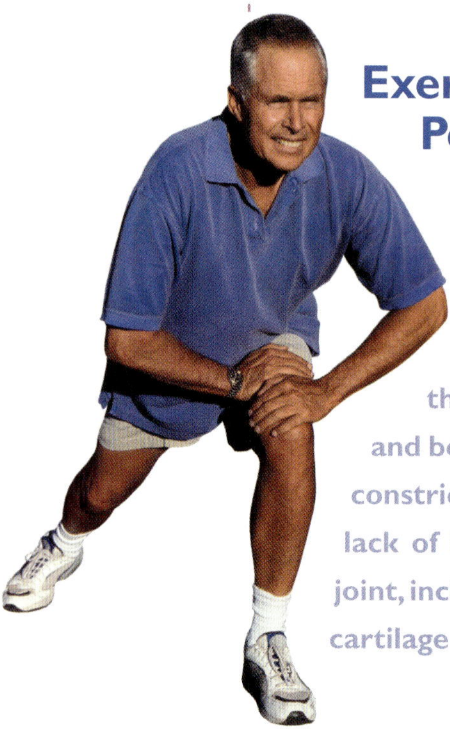

Exercise and Joints: Perfect Together

The well-worn fitness adage "Use it or lose it" certainly applies to your joints. Unless you put them through their paces with regular activity, they lose their strength and resilience and become weaker, stiffer, more painful and constricted. That's because exercise (or the lack of it) affects the health of all parts of a joint, including the bones and the all-important cartilage that covers the ends of them.

Working Out: How Often?

- Try to do stretching (range-of-motion) exercises every day or at least every other day.
- Strengthening exercises should be done every other day, so that muscles can rest between workouts.
- Try to do aerobic exercises for 20 to 30 minutes three times a week.

BONING UP: Bones are dynamic, not static, constantly changing in response to the demands placed on them. Bones are like muscles, growing thicker and stronger in response to a heavier work load.

Experts recommend three types of exercise for arthritis sufferers: stretching (range-of-motion), strength training, and weight-bearing (aerobic) activities like walking. Each works in a different but important way to strengthen and improve joints.

Be flexible

The joint's range of motion—how fully you can bend your knee to pick up a pencil or your grandchild, for example—depends on the flexibility of its supporting cast: the muscles, tendons, and ligaments that surround and protect it. When pain and stiffness discourage people from moving their arthritic joints, the inactivity causes these surrounding tissues to contract—which further limits the joints' movement. Stretching exercises are vital for flexible muscles, tendons, and ligaments, so that range of motion can be maintained and even enhanced.

> "Exercise may be the most effective and inexpensive modality available to achieve optimal outcomes for people with osteoarthritis."
>
> —Marian A. Minor, PT, Ph.D., Rheumatic Disease Clinics of North America, May 1999

Strengthen the supporting cast

The bones of a joint don't operate in isolation. Their ability to move depends on the muscles and tendons that pull on them. Exercises that strengthen muscles and tendons can facilitate movement and help the joints move with less pain. Bulking up the muscle mass around a joint also helps protect the joint in the event of falls or other physical insults.

All people tend to lose muscle mass as they get older, creating a double whammy for older arthritis sufferers: they lose muscle mass "naturally" as they age, and they also lose it because of the inactivity brought on by their condition. This is why muscle-strengthening exercises are valuable for all older people, but especially for those with arthritis.

what the studies show

Recent studies suggest that defects in the portion of bone just beneath a joint's cartilage may play a role in causing osteoarthritis. Weight-bearing exercise is known to stimulate bone growth—it helps to ward off the bone-thinning disorder osteoporosis, for example—and its effect on bone may protect against osteoarthritis, too.

Coddling your cartilage

Smooth movement within a joint depends on the health of its cartilage. (It's the wearing away of cartilage where the bones come together that results in the pain and stiffness of osteoarthritis.) To maximize the health of a joint and its cartilage, the joint must not only move regularly but must actually undergo "repetitive joint loading"—the stress exerted by aerobic, weight-bearing exercises such as walking or jogging.

BONING UP: For every year that you've been out of shape, you need a month or more to get back in shape.

A brief anatomy lesson. Recall that cartilage is not solid like bone, but supple and flexible—contracting and expanding like a sponge each time weight is applied to it. The cartilage in your knee, for example, compresses slightly each time you take a step and then, as you step with your other foot, it expands to return to its resting shape.

The spongy cartilage is filled with and surrounded by synovial fluid, which is soaked up and then wrung out with each step. This soak/squeeze action lubricates the cartilage, preventing it from drying out and becoming stiff. But perhaps even more important, these repetitive stresses also stimulate cartilage growth and repair.

Unlike most tissues, cartilage doesn't have blood vessels that can supply its nourishment. Instead, cartilage must get nutrients from the synovial fluid that bathes it. Only through the repetitive stresses from weight-bearing activities can chondrocytes—the cartilage-making cells—receive the nutrients that enable them to produce more cartilage. If you already have arthritis, weight-bearing exercise can help maintain your remaining cartilage and help stop the disease in its tracks. What's more, maintaining cartilage health through regular weight-bearing exercise may actually help prevent osteoarthritis from occurring in the first place.

In the absence of a cure, exercise is arguably the best available therapy for arthritis of all kinds. The less active you've been until now, the more dramatic the benefits are likely to be.

Small Steps Make A Big Difference

Sixty percent of Americans don't exercise regularly, and 25 percent aren't active at all. In a way, this exercise antipathy is understandable: Intense exercise and its macho slogans ("No pain, no gain," "You've got to feel the burn!") are enough to discourage anyone from lacing on a pair of sneakers and hitting the treadmill or track. Fortunately, the best exercise slogan today is actually a very old one: All things in moderation.

Lifestyle fitness. The value of moderate exercise received publicity in 1995, when the U.S. Centers for Disease Control and Prevention and the American College of Sports Medicine urged Americans to include some form of exercise in their daily lives. The message was that moderate exercise—as little as 30 minutes a day, four times a week—can improve health, and that it could include activities such as walking, biking, gardening, or even housecleaning.

BONING UP: On days when you don't feel motivated, plan on exercising for just five minutes. If you still don't feel like exercising afterward, quit. Most of the time, though, you'll start feeling invigorated and you'll continue.

did you know

You don't have to do all your exercising in one long session. You'll gain nearly the same health benefits by breaking it up into shorter segments throughout the day, whenever you have some spare time.

This "exercise prescription" is amply supported by research showing that moderate activity offers many of the same health benefits previously associated with full-throttle exercise. Consider the results of two such studies:

Researchers at the University of Minnesota observed 12,000 men over a seven-year period. They found that the men who walked or performed comparably demanding exercise for an average of just 20 minutes daily were 37 percent less likely to die from heart disease than men who exercised less than that.

A different group of Minnesota researchers followed some 40,000 postmenopausal women for seven years. Those who regularly participated in moderate exercise such as bowling, golf, gardening, or walking had a 41 percent lower death rate than those who did easier exercise or none at all. Even women who did those activities just once a week had a 29 percent lower mortality rate than those who seldom or never exercised.

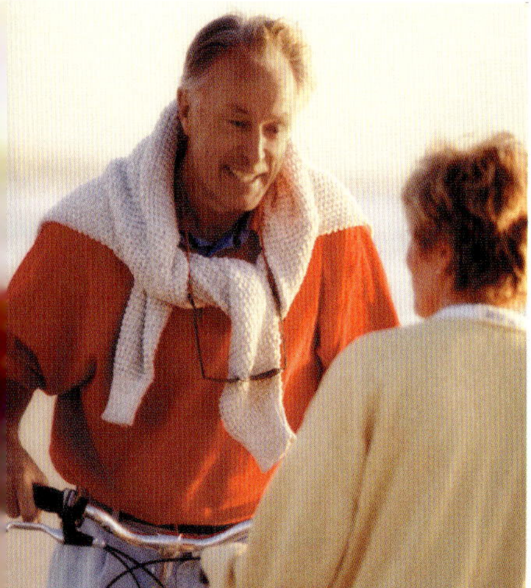

The good news about moderate exercise couldn't come at a better time for people with arthritis. Studies have shown that it's safe for virtually all arthritis patients to engage in moderate exercise—and extremely useful as well: low-impact aerobics, swimming, dancing, walking, and biking are all examples of moderate exercise that can ease joint pain and stiffness while also improving your overall health.

The Essence of Taking Charge

The best way to incorporate exercise into your daily routine is to make it a key piece of your take-charge plan. Most arthritis patients can find some form of exercise that is appropriate—and even fun—for them. And of all possible treatment approaches, exercise may be the one most likely to lead to self-empowerment.

By now, you know how important it is for arthritis patients to embrace the belief that they can control their own destiny. In study after study, self-empowered patients proved most successful in overcoming their symptoms and leading richer, fuller lives. Gaining that mind set involves choosing a long-term goal and then reaching it through a succession of short-term goals. It's a journey that seems tailor-made for exercise.

Exercise builds confidence. Studies have already shown that exercise gives people confidence that they can meet the physical challenges of life—the essence of self-empowerment.

Actions can be specified. A key element in taking charge of arthritis is your take-charge plan (see p.106), in which you list the actions you hope to achieve each week. Exercise is ideal for a take-charge plan, since you can express it as a number of repetitions (12 leg lifts, for example), a distance ("walk one mile"), a length of time ("do stretching exercises for 10 minutes"), or even specify its intensity ("walk 10 minutes on a treadmill set at 3.5 miles per hour").

Keeping score is easy. You know whether you've met your target goal of "two sets of 12 leg lifts on Monday, Wednesday, and Friday."

You can make adjustments. If 12 leg lifts prove too difficult to do, reduce your repetitions to 10.

You can readily build on your success. The take-charge approach is based on gradual progress—achieving small successes each week until you finally achieve a goal that may once have seemed out of reach. A well-planned exercise program follows the same script, with regimens becoming slightly more strenuous from week to week.

Ask the Experts

For most people, exercise is a simple proposition: Put on a pair of sneakers or a swimsuit, start exercising, and sweat. But for arthritis patients who have damaged a joint, strained the supporting ligaments or tendons, or have muscle imbalances, consulting your physician and possibly a physical therapist may be a smarter first move.

Physical therapists are exercise specialists who can work with you to create a program of stretching, strengthening, and aerobic exercises that is tailored to your needs and abilities. You may especially need that kind of advice if your arthritis is severe or if you fell off the exercise wagon a long time ago.

Getting physical. A physical therapist will assess your aerobic capacity, your sense of balance, the flexibility of all your joints, and your muscular strength. Then the therapist will develop a program targeted to areas where you need help—quadriceps-strengthening exercises for knee pain, for example, or swimming to improve aerobic capacity and overall flexibility. Ideally, the choices will include activities you enjoy, so you'll be motivated to stick with the regimen for years to come.

did you know

If pain is your excuse to skip exercise, try a dose of moist heat first. Applying moist heat packs, taking tolerably hot baths or showers, soaking in a hot tub, or swimming in a well-heated pool can help you get moving.

Exercise Carrots: Ways to Keep Moving

- Get a workout partner. If someone is depending on you for his or her exercise, you will be more likely to get up and out instead of hitting your radio's snooze button.
- Log it. Placing a red **X** on a calendar on the days you exercise, or writing about specifics of a workout in a notebook, can turn exercise into a main event in your life.
- Buy a toy. A new heart-rate monitor, fancy leotard, or cool pair of athletic shoes can be all it takes to get you out and about.
- Music makes it. While studies show that people who read or watch television when they work out actually perform with less power and intensity, music has been found to stimulate the feel-good chemicals of the brain, called endorphins.
- Get competitive. Training for an event or competition can prevent boredom.
- Be a morning person. Work out first thing in the A.M. and you'll have gotten your exercise in, no matter how busy your day becomes.
- Combine your workout with work. Bike or walk to work or find ways to do some exercise on your lunch hour.
- Ease up. On your "down" days, do just a few minutes of exercise rather than skipping it completely.

A course of physical therapy generally lasts just a few weeks, although some people may benefit from longer-term care. Therapy sessions usually last less than an hour and may range in frequency from once a week to every day.

The best way to find a physical therapist is to ask your doctor for a referral—and, in fact, some states require it. All physical therapists must be licensed, and some are also certified by the American Board of Physical Therapy Specialists in fields such as geriatrics, neurology, orthopedics, and sports. Physical therapists work in hospitals, clinics, health clubs, cardiac rehabilitation centers, and nursing homes. Some of them even make house calls.

Stretching It: Unlocking the Joints

Of the three types of exercise recommended for arthritis, stretching is the one you should probably do every day. It is the least likely of the three types to cause injury or to aggravate your condition—one reason that some stretching is recommended even during arthritis flares.

Don't be a stiff. Stretching addresses a problem that affects everyone, whether they have arthritis or not: the tendency for muscles, ligaments, tendons, and joints to stiffen with age. Without regular stretching, the average adult's flexibility declines by roughly five percent per decade.

Adding arthritis to the mix makes things considerably worse, since people with the condition are even less likely than others to maintain limber joints. The good news is that inflexible joints can be unlocked—and a conscientious stretching program can help erase decades' worth of accumulated joint tightness.

BONING UP: Stretching exercises to reduce pain are considered a mainstay in the treatment of fibromyalgia, a disease that mainly affects women and is characterized by chronic, generalized musculoskeletal pain.

Why it works. The concept behind stretching (also known as range-of-motion exercises) is simple: When a muscle is pulled slightly beyond its normal length, it gradually adapts to its longer length and increases a joint's range of motion. This improved range

now and then

In 1998, the American College of Sports Medicine expanded the traditional goals of exercise—developing aerobic fitness and muscle strength—to include a third key goal: flexibility. The college urged all Americans to add stretching to their regular exercise program, based on the "growing evidence of its multiple benefits."

caution

Avoid "bounce" stretching—repeated, brief, forceful stretches. They can actually cause damage and increase stiffness.

accounts for most of the benefits of stretching—being able to tie your shoes, work in the garden, or turn your head while driving to see whether a car is in your blind spot.

The ABC's of Stretching

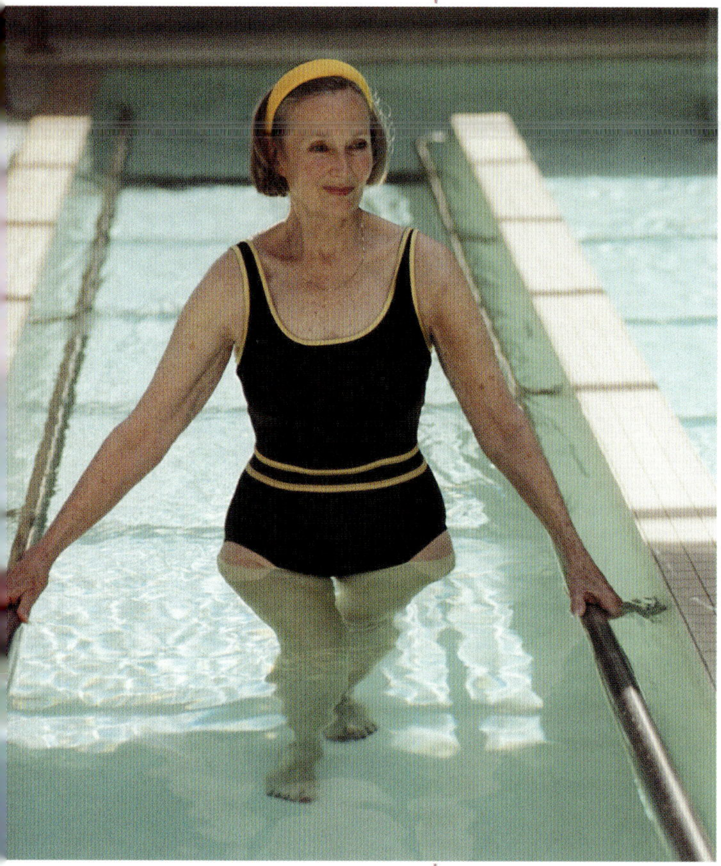

Stretching can be done in several different ways, but one technique—static stretching—is probably safest and is also simple and effective. Static stretching involves easing into a stretch to the point where you begin to feel mild discomfort—never beyond—and then holding that "maximum" position for 10 to 30 seconds. Research has shown that holding a stretch longer than that doesn't provide any additional benefits—and that briefer stretches probably won't do you any good.

Water is an ideal place to stretch, since it supports your limbs and helps minimize stress on them as you put them through their range of motion. Exercising in warm water (between 83 and 90 degrees F.) can be especially useful, since the warmth helps relax muscles and decrease joint pain.

Strength Training: Muscle from Metal

You may well think that strength training is only for young, buffed people in Spandex hefting around barbells that exceed their own body weight. So you may be surprised to learn that older people are the ones who should be flocking to the weight room. The reason? The older people get, the faster they lose muscle strength.

Stretching Do's and Don'ts

- Never stretch a cold muscle; always warm up first. Do your stretching at the end of your exercise routine; or warm up muscles with a slow walk or with a five-or 10-minute stint on the treadmill—then stretch.
- For most stretches you want to be down on the floor so you can relax your body, especially the area that you are stretching. If you don't relax the area you're stretching, your muscles will tighten slightly and you won't make much progress.
- Don't hold your breath while stretching. Your muscles need the oxygen. Exhale as you try to stretch farther.
- Stop if you feel any pain. Pain indicates you're damaging tissues. You should feel the stretch, not pain.
- Form is everything. Don't cheat your stretch by contorting your body or using other joints to compensate for inflexibility.
- If you feel any unusual pains or feel sick in any way, stop and see your physician.

Between the age of 20 and 50, muscle strength in the average American adult dips by only about 10 to 20 percent. But over the next two decades, remaining strength falls by an additional 25 to 30 percent—and plunges even faster after that. Inactivity accounts for much of this muscle loss, so it stands to reason that older people with arthritis become even weaker than other people their age.

Losing more than muscle. As your muscles do a slow fade, it can have serious consequences for your daily life. Many older people have trouble performing everyday tasks such as carrying the laundry, opening windows, or simply getting out of a chair. Muscle loss also weakens the bones, which need stimulation from the muscles to stay strong. And, of course, the inactivity brought on by arthritis weakens the muscles around joints, limiting a person's ability to move and eventually impairing balance.

did you know

If you're a beginning weight lifter or suffer from severe arthritis, you can shed the dumbbells and try new sand-filled nylon weights. They are easier to hold, especially if you have arthritis of the hands, and won't hurt as much if you drop one on your toes or other body part.

Now for the silver lining: Strength training can almost entirely reverse the muscle loss that has occurred over decades. One study, for example, found that 70-year-old men who had engaged in strength training since middle age were just as strong, on average, as 28-year-olds who didn't strength-train. Furthermore, the older people get, the greater their proportional gain from strength training. One study found that frail individuals in their 80s and 90s were able to double or even triple their leg strength after strength-training for just two months, enabling some of them to start walking without a cane.

BONING UP: Holding your breath when strength training can elevate blood pressure to dangerous levels. Olympic weight lifters have been known to drive their BP to 480/320. Instead, breathe out while lifting the weight and breathe in while lowering it.

More muscle, less pain. Strength training has also produced impressive results in studies involving arthritis patients, particularly those with OA of the knee. Almost invariably, the inactivity brought on by OA of the knee causes weakening of the quadriceps muscle, the large muscle in the front of the thigh that runs from the knee to the hip. Exercises that strengthen the quadriceps muscle can produce striking improvements—greatly easing pain and permitting much more movement of the knee joint.

In a study carried out at the State University of New York at Buffalo, 80 people with OA of the knee were put on a three-day-a-week strength-training program. After three months, 90 percent of the participants had less pain, 85 percent had improved the muscle strength around their knees, and 95 percent were better able to perform daily activities. (At the end of this chapter, we describe several exercises that can help you strengthen your quadriceps muscle if OA of the knee is your problem.)

What's more, strength training helps you stay slim because the muscle it builds burns calories faster than fat does, even while you're resting. In general, a strength-training session will use up calories as fast as walking does.

did you know

- Women who worry that strength training may give them a bulky physique can relax. It won't happen—no matter how hard you train—since women have very little testosterone, the hormone that fuels muscle growth. Yet women can build muscle strength as rapidly as men, even after their muscles have attained peak size.
- For some arthritis patients, lifting weights causes pain if the weight is moved through the entire range of motion. Rather than trying to work through the pain, lift the weight through a limited range of motion. You will still experience significant benefit from the lift, and gradually be able to push farther.

Muscles 101

Strength training involves exerting your muscles against resistance—which can be provided by dumbbells, barbells, weight machines, elastic bands, or even your own body weight. Engaging in at least two muscle-strengthening sessions per week will build muscle—and even just one weekly session will slow muscle loss and possibly stop it entirely. The sessions need not be time-consuming: You can obtain substantial benefits from as few as four to six exercises that work the major muscles in the arms, shoulders, chest, back, and legs.

Performing one set of eight to 12 repetitions of a particular strength-training exercise should improve muscle strength and endurance. Interestingly, for the average person, doing multiple sets provides no additional benefits (at least for the first six months) while increasing the risk of injury.

what the studies show

Strength training does more than build muscle. Studies show that it also reduces levels of artery-clogging LDL cholesterol and may actually help to reduce blood pressure.

Strength Training Do's and Don'ts

- Warm up your muscles with a five- or 10-minute aerobic workout on a stair-stepper or treadmill, or take a walk. Your muscles will be better able to lift the load you will be asking them to handle.
- Focus on good form rather than on lifting heavy weight. Don't jerk weights into position with each lift and let them crash back down. Instead, lift and release slowly.
- Tighten the muscle you are working throughout the entire range of motion of a particular exercise, maintaining the tension. This approach recruits more muscle fibers to do the work.
- Try to cover all major muscle groups during each workout.
- Vary your routine. There are more than 200 hundred different types of strength-training exercises. After a couple of weeks, begin substituting new exercises for old ones.
- If you feel pain or odd feelings in your joints while exercising, stop. You may be doing the exercise wrong or using too much weight.
- Gently stretch muscles after a workout.

did you know

If you engage in low-impact aerobic dancing, you can boost the aerobic intensity by increasing the arm movements you make either at or above shoulder level.

Aerobic Exercise: Heavy Breathing Three Times a Week

Exercises that raise your heart rate are considered aerobic. More specifically, aerobic exercise is any activity that uses your large muscles in a repetitive fashion long enough to get your heart beating at 60 to 80 percent of its maximum rate for at least 20, but preferably 30, minutes.

Aerobic exercise—which includes activities like bicycling, walking, swimming, jumping rope, rowing, roller-skating, ice-skating, and cross-country skiing—increases your overall fitness by training your heart and lungs to deliver oxygen more efficiently to the working muscles of the body.

Since people with arthritis tend to be less active and therefore less fit, they usually have a lot to gain from aerobic exercise. Additionally, aerobic exercises that also involve weight bearing, such as walking or jogging, can help to lubricate and nourish the crucially important joint cartilage.

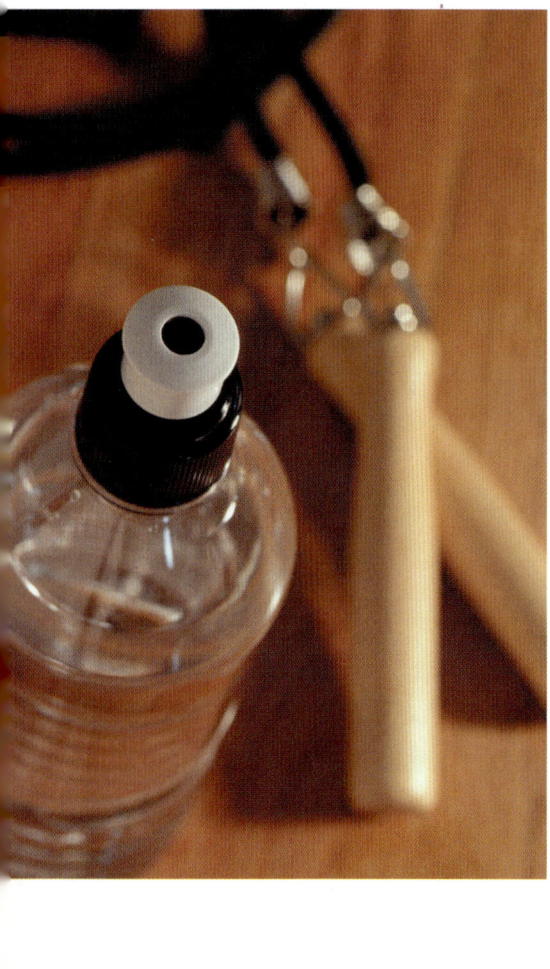

BONING UP: During the first six months of an exercise program, expand the length of your workouts gradually. Increase your sessions by no more than five minutes a month.

Some aerobic exercises do double-duty for arthritis patients, stretching and strengthening the joints. Swimming, for example, is both a good aerobic exercise and ideal for stretching. Walking and dancing are aerobic and also help build strength in both the leg and thigh muscles.

To improve your aerobic capacity, you should exercise at between 60 and 80 percent of the maximum heart rate for your age. This ideal range for aerobic exercising is known as your target heart rate. (See *Calculating Your Heart Rate*, page 244.)

The aerobic exercises generally recommended for

arthritis patients offer a good workout without putting a lot of pressure on your joints. They include walking, biking, swimming, aerobic dancing, and aerobic pool exercises—all of which have been shown to produce definite benefits.

In one study, patients with painful hip or knee OA were randomly assigned to three treatment programs—aerobic walking, aerobic pool exercises, or nonaerobic stretching exercises—for 12 weeks. Both of the aerobic groups showed significant gains in aerobic capacity compared with the stretching group, while all three groups showed similar improvement in joint pain and tenderness. And in case you fear that exercise will send you to the medicine cabinet for pain relief: None of the three groups increased its use of pain medication throughout the study period.

Workout Dropout? Tips to Keep You in Motion

Although many people take the initiative to begin working out, more than half of them quit within three months. All too often, these "workout dropouts" injure themselves by plunging in too aggressively rather than taking things slowly. Fortunately, by taking some basic precautions, you can minimize the risk that an exercise injury will derail your efforts to strengthen your joints.

Get a checkup. If you're over 50, or haven't been physically active for many years, you should see a physician to find out if your heart is up to the rigors of moderate exercise. A doctor's visit is also advisable if you know you have heart disease or one or more risk factors for heart disease, such as hypertension, diabetes, or an elevated cholesterol level.

Even if vigorous exercise is out, you should work with your doctor in choosing stretching or other less-strenuous activity that can still be quite helpful.

Choose your exercises wisely. Whether you design your own exercise program or consult with a physical therapist or other expert, be sure to match your joints with the exercises that

what the studies show

- A study has found that the great majority of older people don't need a stress test, in which heart function is measured as a patient works out on a treadmill. Researchers at Yale University concluded that the risk of heart attack from strenuous exercise has been overstated—and is outweighed by the health benefits that exercise can yield.
- For people with RA and other forms of inflammatory arthritis, aerobic exercise seems to offer a special bonus: reducing joint inflammation. Studies have shown that RA patients who completed aerobic exercise programs had fewer inflamed joints than nonparticipants.

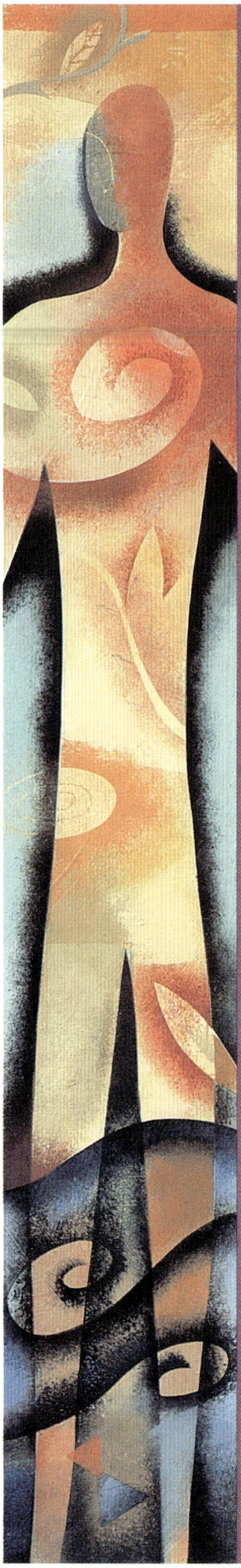

REAL-LIFE MEDICINE

Putting the Moves On Arthritis

Jayne Konrad has nothing against dealing with arthritis as part of a group. In fact, she's the leader of an arthritis support group in the Sacramento, California, area. But when it comes to exercising to ease her pain and stiffness, she prefers to go solo.

Jayne developed osteoarthritis early in life, at around age 25. (Both her parents also developed OA at young ages.) Her hands were severely affected, and her ankles, knees, hips, and neck also gave her problems. Jayne managed to stay active despite her joint pain: "I pretty much kept up because I was young enough to," says Jayne. "During my 30s and 40s I raised two children, I rode horses, I raised, bred, and showed dogs, I ran, I did everything."

But starting about 10 years ago, Jayne's condition worsened. She sometimes required a walker and was classified as disabled. Three years ago she was told she had rheumatoid arthritis as well. "Finally, I started saying, 'I've got to do something about this,'" Jayne recalls. So she became an exerciser.

"For about two years I went to a community center that offered an exercise program for older people," said Jayne, who is 62 years old. "But I found that I only exercised for about 20 minutes of the hour-long class. I couldn't exercise lying on the floor, since I wasn't able to get back up again. And the instructor did the same routines every day—you could guess what she was going to say before she even said it."

So Jayne created her own exercise program, and it has made all the difference. She essentially exercises from the minute she wakes up in the morning until a couple of hours before she goes to bed. ("You shouldn't exercise right before you go to bed or else you'll have trouble falling to sleep," she warns.)

"I start before I even get out of bed, first moving my feet and then working my way up the body," she says. "I pull my knees up and lower them, back and forth, then I stretch my arms and hands and wrists. Then I sit on the side of the bed and do more exercises, straightening and bending my knees." Jayne continues doing exercises after getting up, including what she describes as "pushups against the wall" to stretch her calf muscles.

In the afternoon comes another

workout. "I put on music, quite often jazz, and dance in my living room. I just make things up as I go along as I dance and stretch," says Jayne. Later in the afternoon comes walking for 30 or 45 minutes most every day. In the summer Jayne also uses the outdoor pool available in the park, as well as a Jacuzzi. But she's most proud of the exercising she does while doing other things.

"There are always things you can do just in the course of a normal day, without rowing machines or any other apparatus," says Jayne. "Standing in line at the grocery store, you can bend your knees up and down, strengthening your thigh muscles as you're waiting to check out and pay the bill.

"I also have spongy rubber balls in different places around the house," explains Jayne. "So if I'm watching TV or working at my computer, I'm also squeezing the ball to exercise my hands and fingers, and also turning my ankles first one way, then another. You're sitting there, but you're also doing something useful. If you keep it up, then little by little you can progress further and further."

"I start exercising before I even get out of bed," says Jayne.

Jayne readily lists the changes that exercising has made in her life. For someone with debilitating arthritis, attaining victories like these can evoke hallelujahs. "I can get up from a seated position now without having to pull myself up—that's a major accomplishment," she says. "I no longer have to walk in baby steps anymore but now I can take normal steps—a big, big improvement. And you know those cookies that you slice and bake? I'm able to slice them now, and until recently I couldn't."

For a zealous basketball fan like Jayne, having arthritis was especially frustrating when she attended games, so perhaps the most notable change that has resulted from her exercise routine is evident when she attends Sacramento Kings games at Arco Arena. "I have season tickets and attend the games with my daughter's family," says Jayne. "Our seats are in the upper deck, a long way up. Two years ago I couldn't climb those stairs, and now I can."

Calculating Your Heart Rate

To calculate your maximum heart rate, do the following:

1. Subtract your age from 220. For example, if you're 55 years old, you're maximum heart rate would be 220 – 55 = 165 beats per minute.

2. Calculate the lower end of your target heart rate by taking 60 percent of 165, which equals 99.

3. Calculate the upper limit of your target heart rate by taking 80 percent of 165, which equals 132.

So, at age 55, your target heart range while exercising should be between 99 and 132 beats per minute. To improve your aerobic capacity, you should try to work out within your target heart range for 20 to 30 minutes three times per week.

You can monitor your heart rate by finding your pulse. Place your fingertips on the palm side of your wrist or lay them lightly against the side of your larynx (voice box), count the pulses for 15 seconds, and then multiply this number by four to get your pulse rate in beats per minute.

caution

Rest is certainly advisable if you've overdone things or if you're having a flare-up of joint pain (although even then you should probably do some gentle stretching exercises). But avoid the temptation to rest your joints for long periods of time, since the inactivity may actually increase pain and stiffness. Remember that not exercising poses far more risk to arthritic joints than doing proper exercises.

are most appropriate for them. If you have an arthritic shoulder, for example, include shoulder-stretching exercises but avoid strenuous weight lifting. If your knees are painful, then wind sprints are probably not in your future. By showing common sense in the exercises you choose, you can ensure that your program will improve your arthritis without causing injuries.

Warm up. Muscles are somewhat like taffy: As they warm up, they become more pliant—easier to stretch and less likely to tear. So warming up prior to a workout can be quite important for avoiding injuries, but too many people don't take the time to do it. A good warmup usually takes seven to 10 minutes—and even longer if in the past you've injured yourself while exercising. The idea is to raise your body temperature, elevate your heart rate, and loosen up the muscles and joints so they can withstand the stresses they'll soon be confronting. Good ways to warm up include pedaling on a stationary bike, moderately fast walking, or jogging in place.

Stretch. Stretching is not only a useful prelude to exercise but is also a vital form of exercise in its own right for people with arthritis. Contrary to standard wisdom, researchers have found that stretching before a workout does not decrease the risk of injury, but it does help reduce the pain and discomfort that can occur when stiff joints are made to move. As noted above, people with arthritis should do stretching exercise every day or at least every other day. But when stretching precedes other types of exercise, one continuous 15-to 30-second stretch should suffice for most muscle groups.

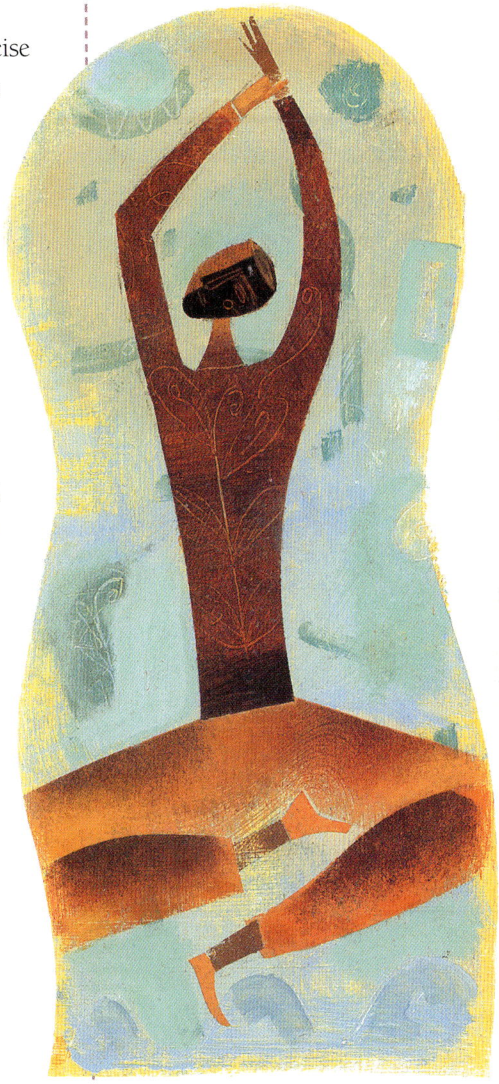

Ease into it. For the first two weeks, maintain an easy, relaxed pace. Exercise for no more than 10 or 20 minutes at a time and no more than three or four times a week. You should expect a little muscle soreness when you embark on any exercise program

Soften the impact. Arthritis patients should be especially careful to protect sensitive joints from unaccustomed jolts. So you should limit yourself to low-impact exercises such as walking, biking, or swimming, and try to work out on soft, smooth surfaces such as grass, dirt, or cushioned surfaces in a gym.

In addition, proper footwear can be a big help in defusing the shocks of repeated impacts. Buy high-quality running or walking shoes from a good athletic shoe store that employs knowledgeable salespeople. You want shoes that are suited to your particular feet, so ask whether your feet underpronate (usually meaning you have high arches and need good arch support) or overpronate (meaning you probably have flat-feet and need a well-cushioned sole). Replace your shoes as soon as they seem to have lost some cushioning ability—even if the tread still looks new.

To further muffle the pounding, consider buying cushioned insoles for your shoes. One study found that wearing such

Splint It!

When something—too much exercise, say—suddenly turns up the volume on your joint pain, there is a time-proven way of lowering it: rest. And one of the oldest, most effective ways of doing that is with a splint.

New approaches to an old remedy. Today's splints are lighter and sleeker than those of the past and made of plastic or a combination of plastic and rubber. They can be purchased over-the-counter or custom-fitted, usually by an occupational therapist. One of the simplest splints is a slip-on variety used to immobilize the joints of the fingers. (A variation is the silver-ring splint, which allows limited movement of the finger joints). Splints can also be fitted to many other joints as well, such as the wrist or elbow.

Splints are never worn permanently, but instead are designed to be easily put on and taken off as needed. Sometimes splints are worn during the day, but your doctor may recommend that you wear it only at night.

insoles while walking can decrease the shock measured at the knee by nearly 50 percent.

Heed your senses. You can expect some muscle soreness when you first start an exercise program. But don't continue exercising if joint pain worsens, and stay tuned for other warning signs that you've overdone it, including:

- Muscle or joint pain that lasts more than two hours after you've stopped exercising
- Unusually severe fatigue
- Increased muscle weakness
- Decreased range of motion of one or more joints
- Increased joint swelling

Water power. You need water to replace fluids you lose through perspiration and to reduce the risk of muscle cramps. Try to drink two glasses of water two hours before you exercise, an additional glass every 20 minutes while you're exercising, and another glass or two within the hour after you stop exercising.

Cool down. Suddenly stopping exercise can sharply reduce blood pressure, causing fainting or even a heart attack. So, just as you took time to warm up when you started, end each session with a cooldown period in which you spend a few minutes doing stretches and slow walking or gentle calisthenics.

BONING UP: Try to exercise when joints are least likely to feel stiff or fatigued, perhaps in the late morning or early afternoon.

The Top 20: Exercises That Strengthen and Stretch

Some exercises can increase flexibility and strengthen the muscles and other tissues that bend the joint. Most of the ones described below fall into this two-for-one category.

These exercises can be done daily. Start in gradually, doing two or three repetitions of each exercise; then slowly increase your number of repetitions until, for each exercise, you can do three sets of 10 repetitions (30 repetitions in all) in one session.

Good Moves for the Knees

Quad tighteners

- Lie on your back with your legs comfortably bent at the knee, and prop yourself up with your forearms.
- Extend one leg until it's straight, and then tighten the thigh muscle of your extended leg; note that this action should push the back of your knee down to the floor. Then switch legs and repeat to complete one repetition.

Foot lifts

- Place a firm pillow under one knee and lie flat on your back. (Bend your other leg comfortably at the knee, keeping the foot on the floor.)
- Without moving your knee off the pillow, slowly raise your

what the studies show

Women who ate a moderately low-calorie diet and did either strength training or aerobic exercise lost more weight than women who just dieted. But those women who split their workout time between aerobic exercise and strength training lost the most weight of all.

Better Biomechanics

Although exercise can help your joints and arthritis, poor posture and biomechanics can cancel out that good medicine. Here are some suggestions that can take the strain out of daily tasks:

- If you have arthritis of the hands, use an electric can opener rather than a manual model. What's more, don't hold objects in a tight grip for extended periods. When holding anything, flex your fingers frequently.
- If reaching up hurts your shoulder, place frequently used items on lower shelves.
- Use good posture. It places the least stress on your joints.
- Use the largest joint possible to accomplish any task. Carry a shoulderbag rather than a clutch purse, because your shoulder joint is larger than your finger joints.
- Try to keep your joints extended rather than bent.
- Try not to stay in one position for a long period of time.
- For RA patients, look for reach-and-grab items and extended shoehorns that are easier on inflamed joints.

foot until your leg is straight and then gently lower your foot to the floor. Switch legs and repeat.

Extend and flex

- Sit up straight in a chair with both feet flat on the floor.
- Slowly straighten one leg so that it's parallel to the floor, holding that position for three to five seconds.
- Bend your knee and slowly return your foot to the floor. Repeat with the other leg.

Reach for the stars

- Lie on your back with one leg comfortably bent at the knee and the other extended as straight as possible on the floor.
- Bend the knee of the straight leg, bringing it as far toward your chest as you can.
- Straighten that leg, making sure to push out with your heel, so that your foot points directly upward.

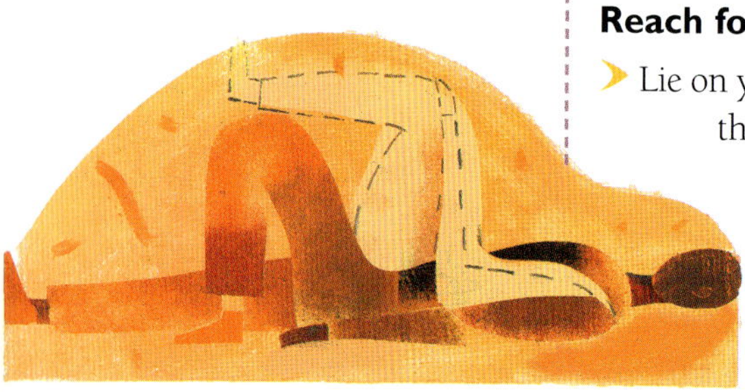

- Bend the knee back toward your chest and lower the leg to the floor.
- Repeat again with the same leg, but this time push your leg out at a different angle. Repeat three to five times, extending your leg at a different angle each time. Then do the same routine with the other leg.

Quad builder

- Lie on your back with one leg bent and the other flat on the floor.
- Flex the foot of the flat leg (i.e., point your toes back toward your head), tighten your knee so the leg is straight, then lift that leg until your foot is two feet off the floor.
- Count slowly to five, then lower the leg slowly, touching the floor with your calf first. Repeat with your other leg.

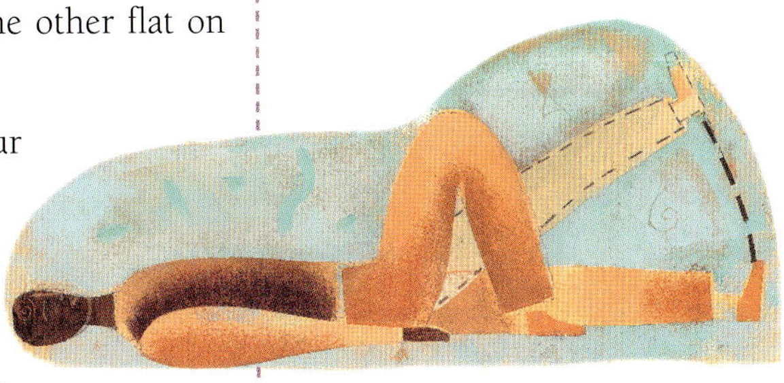

Medicine for the Hips

Side leg lifts

- With your head resting on your arm, lie on your side with the leg you want to exercise on top. (Bend your bottom leg slightly to maintain balance.)
- Being careful to keep your top leg straight and without moving it forward, lift it about two feet off the floor and then slowly lower it. Repeat with the other leg.

Hip rolls

- Lie on your back and extend both legs.
- Rotate one leg inward, then rotate it outward. Repeat with the other leg.

Thigh lifts

- Sit in a chair with both of your feet flat on the floor.
- Raise the knee of your affected leg as high as possible, then slowly lower it.

Help for the Neck

Stare down

- Looking straight ahead with your chin slightly dropped, bend your head forward, keeping your chin tucked in.
- Straighten your head but don't bend it backward.

Arthritis Profile

Theodore Roosevelt, Jr.

His father led the famous charge up San Juan Hill during the Spanish-American War and later became president. But Theodore Roosevelt, Jr. also knew how to take charge: Despite suffering from severe osteoarthritis of the hip, Brigadier General Roosevelt led his troops ashore during the Normandy Invasion—the only general to land with the first assault wave.

On D-Day—June 6, 1944—Roosevelt and his forces landed on Utah Beach. The landing crafts arrived nearly a mile south of their intended target, prompting Roosevelt to tell his men, "We're going to start the war from right here."

For the rest of D-Day—armed with only a pistol, walking with a cane due to his arthritis, and while under constant enemy fire—Roosevelt repeatedly led groups of his men over a sea wall to positions inland. General Omar N. Bradley, commander of the overall amphibious operation, would later describe this as the single bravest action he had ever witnessed.

In a letter to his wife on the eve of the invasion, Roosevelt had written: "I go in with the assault wave and hit the beach at H-Hour. I'm doing it because it's the way I can contribute most. It steadies the young men to see me plodding along with my cane."

For his "valor and courage," Roosevelt was awarded the Congressional Medal of Honor, the nation's highest military award.

Look both ways

- Begin by looking straight ahead, with chin dropped slightly.
- Turn your head and look over your left shoulder.
- Then turn it so you're looking over your right shoulder.

Tick tock

- Look straight ahead with your chin slightly dropped.
- As you continue staring straight ahead, bend your head sideways so that your ear moves toward your shoulder. (Don't lift your shoulder toward your ear.)
- Bend your head to the other side.

Stronger Shoulders and Elbows

Shoulder touch

- Sit or stand with your arms at your sides, palms facing backward.
- Lift both arms forward to shoulder level with both palms facing down.
- Turn your palms up, and touch your fingertips to your shoulders, allowing your elbows to drop.
- Straighten arms at shoulder level, turning palms down.
- Lower your arms slowly, first to your side and behind your back, and then touch your palms together.

Shoulder circle

- Make sure both of your shoulders are relaxed as you look straight ahead.
- Roll both shoulders in circular movements—forward, up, backward, and down.

Touch down

- Sit on a stool or other hard surface with your back straight, your feet flat on the floor, and your hands on your knees.
- Touch your stomach with your hands, keeping your elbows out to the side.
- With elbows extended out to the sides, touch your shoulders, then touch behind your head.
- Stretch both arms upward with your palms facing each other, then lower your arms back to your knees.

A Limber Back

Pelvic tilt

- Lie on your back, knees bent, and feet flat on the floor.
- Press your back against the floor as you tighten your stomach. Hold this position for a count of 10, then relax.

Body curl

- As you flatten your back against the floor in the pelvic tilt position above, slowly bring your knees toward your chest, using your hands to pull your knees even closer. Hold this position for a count of 10, with your knees slightly separated as you do so.
- Slowly allow your feet to return to the floor.

did you know

Pain and stiffness in one joint often leads to problems in another. The ankle, for example, is rarely affected by osteoarthritis, but people with OA of the knee often develop ankles that are weak and have limited motion. The pain in their knee has caused them to walk more gingerly, and with less weight placed on the foot, the calf muscle grows weak and the ankle becomes stiff. For similar reasons, OA of the knee quite often leads to impaired hip motion as well—and vice versa.

Leg slides

- Starting in the pelvic-tilt position, slowly slide one foot away from you until your leg is straightened.
- Slowly pull it back to the bent-knee position, keeping your back pressed to the floor the entire time. Repeat with the other foot.

Curl and slide

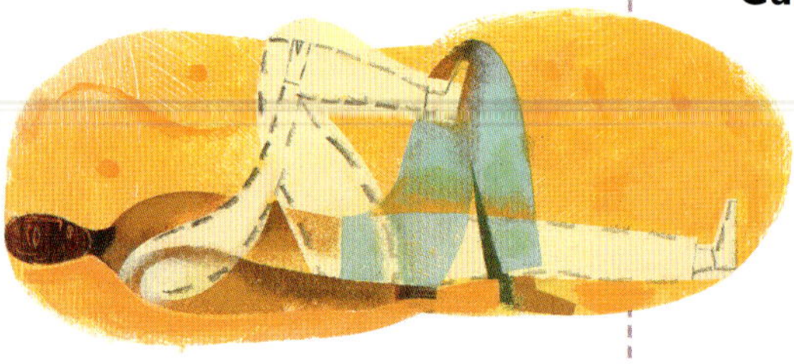

- Lie on your back with your knees bent.
- Bring one knee toward your chest and hold it with both of your hands.
- With your back pressed to the floor, slowly slide your other foot along the floor until that leg is straight.
- With your back still pressed against the floor, slowly slide that leg back until it returns to the bent-knee position. Then switch legs and repeat.

The Buddha

- Sitting with your legs crossed in front of you, hold your feet with your hands.
- Slowly lean forward, moving your face toward the floor. Don't jerk or bob.

Chair bend

- Sit up straight in a chair, with your feet flat and your hands on your hips.
- Look directly ahead, and bend your trunk to one side.
- Return to the sitting-up-straight position, bend over to the other side, and then return to sitting up straight.

Reduce the Stress, Reduce the Pain

Exercise is useful not just for its ability to help nurture cartilage and peel off the pounds, but for its well-advertised benefit of short-circuiting stress. Stress can be a big problem for arthritis patients, increasing sensitivity to pain, tightening the muscles around joints, and hindering movement.

Taking a Load Off

Although exercise is the best way to protect your joints, assistive devices can take the pressure off stiff joints.

The story of cane. Anyone who walks with a limp should consider using a cane; it protects the joints by taking weight off of them and is helpful during a flare-up. Proper use of a cane can relieve pressure on the hip joint by up to 50 percent.

Bath and kitchen tips. Elevated toilet seats with handles and bath benches for the tub can take stress off joints. In the kitchen special knives with **L**-shaped handles, cutting boards that hold foods firmly in place, and electric can openers and jar openers can help arthritis sufferers.

Many studies have shown that regular exercise reduces anxiety, muscle tension, and blood pressure—three key measures of stress—for at least several hours and possibly much longer. Two exercise regimens in particular—yoga and tai chi—may be especially useful for arthritis patients who want to quell anxiety and pain.

Tai Chi: Ballet in Slow Motion

This ancient Chinese discipline could actually serve as a complete fitness program, since its graceful, fluid movements manage to combine the three forms of exercise that lend a helping hand to arthritis patients: strength training, stretching, and aerobic exercise. Several studies have shown that tai chi helps people improve or maintain strength, joint flexibility, and balance, and can also boost aerobic capacity. But in addition, tai chi promotes a sense of well-being and relaxation that arthritis patients should find especially helpful.

BONING UP: **Tai chi doesn't seem to trigger rheumatoid arthritis symptoms. Researchers taught 20 people with RA a tai chi routine and supervised two hour-long sessions a week for 10 weeks. None of the participants experienced any aggravation of symptoms.**

what the studies show

Volunteers between 58 and 70 years old were asked to practice tai chi five days a week. After one year, volunteers experienced 15 to 20 percent improvement in both aerobic capacity and knee strength.

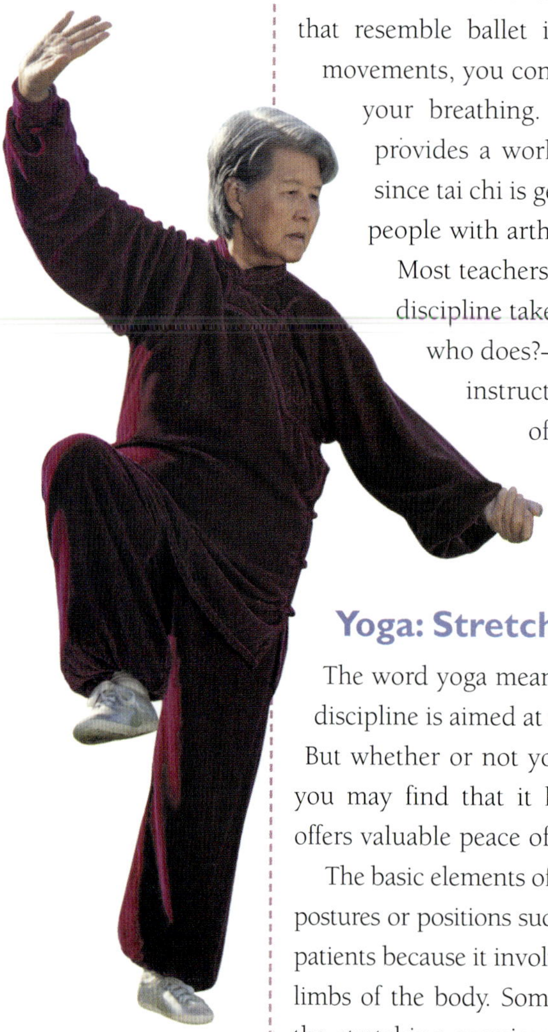

Tai chi consists of a series of movements, known as "forms," that resemble ballet in slow motion. As you perform these movements, you concentrate intently on both the motion and your breathing. The combination of these movements provides a workout for all the limbs and muscles. And since tai chi is gentle and low impact, it's ideally suited for people with arthritis—OA or RA.

Most teachers of tai chi believe that truly mastering the discipline takes a lifetime. If you don't have that long—who does?—take several classes with an experienced instructor. Alternatively, tai chi classes may be offered by your local "Y" or by health clubs, martial-arts schools, and community centers. You can also buy or rent videos that instruct you in tai chi.

Yoga: Stretch Yourself Healthy

The word yoga means "union" and the practice of this Hindu discipline is aimed at uniting the body and mind with the soul. But whether or not you embrace the mystical aspects of yoga, you may find that it helps to relieve arthritis symptoms and offers valuable peace of mind.

The basic elements of yoga are controlled breathing and various postures or positions such as the lotus position. Yoga helps arthritis patients because it involves stretching, extending, and relaxing the limbs of the body. Some yoga positions are virtually identical to the stretching exercises that physical therapists recommend for arthritis patients. Others help to strengthen the muscles, tendons, and ligaments that surround the joint. And most all of them help to reduce stress and create a feeling of relaxation.

For best results with yoga, you should practice it regularly, for 45 minutes or an hour a day if possible. If you can't spare that much time, shorter daily sessions lasting 15 minutes or so are preferable to longer sessions that you do just once or twice a week.

The best way to learn yoga is in a class with a qualified, experienced instructor. Your local "Y" or community center probably offers an introductory course, and videos are also available.

caution

Beware of yoga instructors or courses that make extravagant claims about health benefits obtainable from yoga. The best programs are those that begin with the simplest and safest positions and then become gradually more rigorous.

The Final Word

If you've followed most of the advice in the previous 254 pages, then you may be wondering when you will begin to feel better. Perhaps you already do, but some more unlucky souls may feel disappointed that all this self-empowerment stuff hasn't made a difference in their life.

Patience, patience. Our advice is just wait a little longer. As you follow the take-charge approach, remember that only you can provide the most important ingredient for success: patience. You may well be in pain and your joints probably feel stiff and creaky. Above all, you want to feel better. You can, but it may take time.

In all likelihood, your arthritis developed over the course of many years. Just as it takes time to break a bad habit, it may take awhile—perhaps several months of effort on your part—before you sense that your take-charge efforts have started to turn things around and that you have gained control of your condition.

In addition to patience, the other ingredient that you must provide is perseverance. No arthritis treatment will help all people, but everyone should be able to find a particular therapy, or combination of therapies, that will prove helpful. You may not find it immediately, but you owe it to yourself to keep trying.

Recall the example of Gloria Baswell (on page 158). During the course of several years, she tried virtually all arthritis drugs to treat her rheumatoid arthritis. Through it all she remained patient and persevered, and she finally found an experimental drug that has made all the difference for her.

Gloria also did something else crucial to taking charge: she put great emphasis on informing herself about her disease and treatment options. Medical knowledge is never static—and, in the case of arthritis, major advances have occurred over just the past few years. No time is a good time to develop arthritis, but with recent medical advances and the proven effectiveness of the take-charge approach, people with arthritis can now live more fulfilling, less painful lives than at any time ever. We've come a long way in successfully managing arthritis, and the best may be yet to come.

Organizations for Patients and Professionals

Academy for Guided Imagery

P.O. Box 2070
Mill Valley, CA 94942
800-726-2070
www.heahthy.net/agi

Provides audio tapes on practicing guided imagery and referrals to guided-imagery practitioners in your area.

The American Academy of Medical Acupuncture

5820 Wilshire Blvd., Suite 500
Los Angeles, CA 90036
323-937-5514
800-521-2262

Maintains a directory of members, who are medical doctors and doctors of osteopathy who have completed a training program in acupuncture.

American Chronic Pain Association

P.O. Box 850
Rocklin, CA 95677
916-632-0922
www.http://members.tripod.com/~Widdy/ACPA.html

Provides information on dealing with chronic pain in a positive way and to participate in self-help group activities offered through its 800 affiliated chapters worldwide.

American Chiropractic Association

1701 Clarendon Blvd.
Arlington, VA 22209
800-986-4636
www.amerchiro.org

Offers information on chiropractic and can refer you to a chiropractor in your area.

American College of Rheumatology

60 Executive Park South, Suite 150
Atlanta, GA 30329
404-633-3777
www.rheumatology.org

Offers a list of rheumatologists, physical therapists, and occupational therapists in your area.

American Holistic Medical Association

6728 Old McLean Village Drive
McLean VA 22101
703-556-9327
www.holisticmedicine.org

Provides referrals to medical doctors and doctors of osteopathy in your area who combine alternative and conventional therapies in their practice.

American Massage Therapy Association

820 Davis St., Suite 100
Evanston, IL 60201-4444
847-864-0123
www.amtamassage.org

Represents more than 42,000 massage therapists worldwide and can refer you to a massage therapist in your area.

The American Occupational Therapy Association

4720 Montgomery Lane
P.O. Box 31220
Bethesda, MD 20824-1220
301-652-2682
www.aota.org

American Osteopathic Association

142 East Ontario St.
Chicago, IL 60611
800-621-1773
www.aoa-net.org

Provides information on osteopathic medicine and can provide referrals to osteopathic doctors who specialize in rheumatology.

The American Physical Therapy Association

111 North Fairfax St.
Alexandria, VA 22314
www.apta.org

American Self-Help Clearinghouse

St. Clare's Hospital
Denville, NJ 07834-2995
973-326-6789
www.selfhelpgroups.org

Contact the clearinghouse to find national groups for arthritic disorders and self-help clearinghouses in your area.

Arthritis Foundation

1330 West Peachtree St.
Atlanta, GA 30309
800-283-7800 (for automated information on arthritis available 24 hours a day)
404-872-7100 (or call your local chapter, listed in the phone book)
www.arthritis.org

Provides information about all forms of arthritis. Local chapters offer the Arthritis Self-Help Course referred to in this book, plus other programs such as People with Arthritis Can Exercise (PACE).

The Arthritis Society

393 University Avenue, Suite 1700
Toronto, Ontario M5G 1E6
Canada
416-979-3353
800-321-1433 (usable in Canada only)
www.arthritis.ca

The Canadian equivalent of the Arthritis Foundation, the society provides information about all types of arthritis and the Society's Self-Management Program, offered by the society's provincial divisions and similar to the Arthritis Foundation's self-help course.

Fibromyalgia Network

P.O. Box 31750
Tucson, AZ 85751-1750
800-853-2929
www.fmnetnews.com

Offers educational materials on fibromyalgia and chronic fatigue syndrome.

The Herb Research Foundation

1007 Pearl St., Suite 200
Boulder, CO 80302
303-449-2265
800-748-2617
www.herbs.org/index.html

Offers more than 200 information packets on herbs and specific health conditions.

Lupus Foundation of America

1300 Piccard Drive, Suite 200
Rockville, MD 20850-4303
301-670-9292
800-558-0121
www.lupus.org

Provides information about lupus and the location of the nearest local chapter of the organization.

Lyme Disease Foundation

One Financial Plaza, 18th Floor
Hartford, CT 06103-2610
860-525-2000
800-886-LYME (24-hour hotline)
www.lyme.org

Offers information on Lyme disease and other tickborne diseases.

The Mind-Body Medical Institute

Division of Behavioral Medicine
Beth Israel Deaconess Medical Center
110 Francis St.
Boston, MA 02215
617-632-9530
800-378-6857
www.mindbody.harvard.edu

Offers information about mind-body research and can refer you to a mind-body program in your area.

National Certification Commission for Acupuncture and Oriental Medicine

11 Canal Center Plaza, Suite 330
Alexandria, VA 22314
703-548-9004
www.nccaom.org

This organization certifies acupuncturists and has a directory of practitioners.

National Organization for Rare Disorders (NORD)

P.O. Box 8923
New Fairfield, CT 06812-8923
203-746-6518
800-999-6673
www.rarediseases.org

Patients with psoriatic arthritis, polymyositis, and other relatively rare forms of arthritis can contact NORD for information and additional resources.

Progoff Intensive Journal Program for Self-Development

Dialogue House Associates
80 E. 11th St., Suite 305
New York, NY 10003
212-673-5880
800-221-5844
www.intensivejournal.org

Recent research shows that writing about stressful experiences improves the symptoms of arthritis patients, and participating in this program may help you do that.

Spondylitis Association of America

P.O. Box 5872
Sherman Oaks, CA 91413
800-777-8189
www.spondylitis.com

SSA offers a variety of information about ankylosing spondylitis, including pamphlets and exercise videos and tapes.

Stress Reduction Clinic

Center for Mindfulness in Medicine, Health Care, and Society
University of Massachusetts Medical Center
55 Lake Avenue North
Worcester, MA 01655
508-856-2656
www.umassmed.edu/cfm

Provides information about stress reduction and referrals to a stress-reduction program in your area.

Government Organizations

Combined Health Information Database (CHID)

www.chid.nih.gov
e-mail: chid@aerie.com

A reference tool for health professionals and the general public, CHID pools data from several federal health agencies and offers summaries of thousands of journal articles and patient-education materials on arthritis and 17 other health topics.

National Arthritis and Musculoskeletal and Skin Diseases Information Clearinghouse

National Institutes of Health
1 AMS Circle
Bethesda, MD 20892-3675
301-495-4484
877-22-NIAMS (toll free)
www.nih.gov/niams/

A public service of the National Institute of Arthritis and Musculoskeletal and Skin Diseases, the clearinghouse offers many publications on arthritis, including useful information packages such as "Arthritis and Diet" and "Arthritis and Exercise." Call NIAMS Fast Facts (301-881-2731) for health information available by fax 24 hours a day.

National Center for Complementary and Alternative Medicine Clearinghouse

P.O. Box 8218
Silver Spring, MD 20907-8218
888-644-6226 (toll-free)
www.nccam.nih.gov

Offers information on alternative-medicine research into arthritis as well as other health problems.

National Library of Medicine

www.nlm.nih.gov

You can search the National Library of Medicine's MEDLINE database and view abstracts of journal articles free of charge; full-text copies require a fee.

Internet Resources

Rheuma21st

www.rheuma21st.com/index.html

This "Internet journal," which reports on important developments in rheumatology, is aimed at researchers and clinicians but may also be informative for arthritis patients.

About.com

www.about.com

allHealth

www.allhealth.com

America's Doctor

www.americasdoctor.com

InteliHealth

www.intelihealth.com

MediConsult

www.mediconsult.com

The National Council Against Health Fraud

www.ncahf.org

onHealth

www.onhealth.com

Quackwatch

www.quackwatch.com

webMD

www.webmd.com

A

B

C

E

O

P

Q

R

S

T

U

V

W

X

Y

Credits

Photo

4-5: Photodisc. 10: Photodisc. 14: Spinning Egg Design. 17: Photo Alto. 28: Photodisc. 35: Photo Alto. 41: Stock Market. 42: Photodisc. 52: Stock Market. 66: Photodisc. 81: Photo Alto. 84: Photodisc. 90: Photodisc. 101: Comstock. 105: Comstock. 112: Corbis. 114: Photodisc. 120: Eyewire. 134: Photodisc. 138: Dan Potash. 144: Comstock. 149: Comstock. 154: Eyewire. 160: Eyewire. 170: Photodisc. 174: Corbis. 191: Photodisc. 198: Corbis. 201: Photodisc. 208: Photodisc. 210: Photodisc. 214: Dynamic Graphics. 218: Digital Stock. 221: Eyewire. 223: Photodisc. 226: Photodisc. 232: Stock Market. 236: Eyewire. 240: Photodisc. 254: Photodisc.

Illustration

7, 12, 13, 18, 21, 30, 58, 61, 71, 74, 92, 97, 116, 124, 126, 136, 158, 165, 174, 179, 187, 201, 206, 216, 226, 242, 245,248, 249, 252: Linda Frichtell. 33: Hugo Cruz. 39, 47: Articulate Graphics.

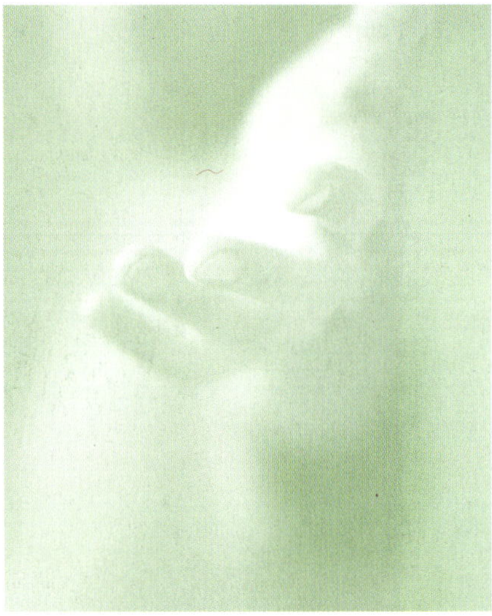